THE GREAT AMERICAN HEALTHCARE BILLING SCAM

Rudi Bester

Memory Trees Corporation 501(c)3

ISBN-13: 9798842181599
ISBN-10: 1477123456

Cover design by: Art Painter
Library of Congress Control Number: 2018675309
Printed in the United States of America

*Dedicated to my family, who were there and waiting for me,
when I awoke from surgery.*

I love you guys!

"And so our goal on health care is, if we can get, instead of health care costs going up 6 percent a year, it's going up at the level of inflation, maybe just slightly above inflation, we've made huge progress. And by the way, that is the single most important thing we could do in terms of reducing our deficit. That's why we did it."

BARACK OBAMA

CONTENTS

INTRODUCTION

I live near a magnificent, luxury beachfront hotel, called Breaker's Resort, located in Palm Beach Island, Florida.

This stunning resort complex charges about $2,000 per night, for an "Atlantic Guest Room with Oceanfront View".

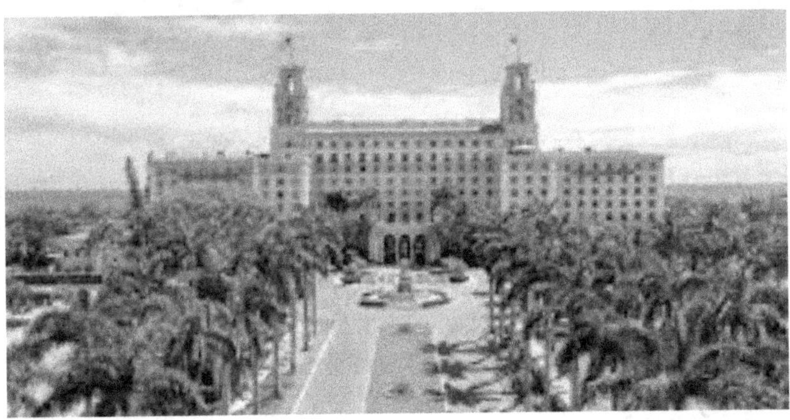

My local hospital, also near my home - and only a few miles from the Breaker's Resort - charges about $3,200 per night for a private room.

During April 2022, I had the privilege of being accommodated in a basic hospital room - without an oceanfront view - for a few nights.

I have not yet splurged on an overnight stay at the Breaker's.

But it is probably safe to assume that the daily rate would include cleaning the room, making the bed, replacing used toiletries, etc.?

At my local medical center, they did not clean the room or change the bedding daily. The room was not very luxurious, but it did feature a few pieces of expensive equipment, like a motorized bed, and machines that beep and feature blinking LEDs.

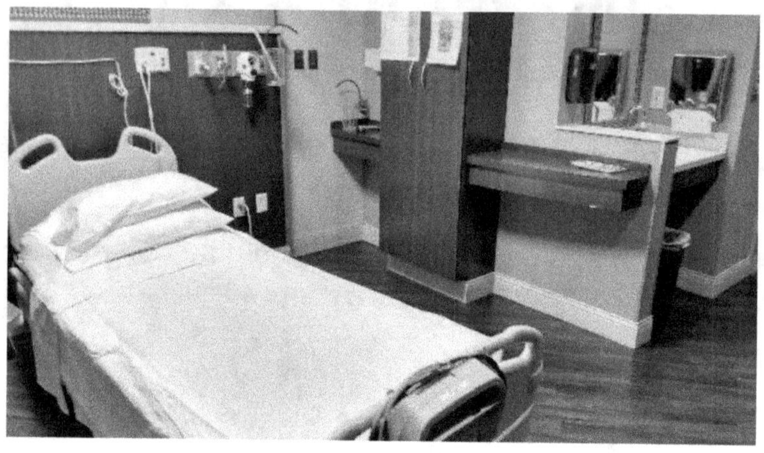

At the Breaker's, in-room food and beverage services would likely be available 24/7, but obviously for quite high, additional fees, I am sure.

I do not know what the additional costs would be for food and beverages at my local hospital, because I was not served, nor offered anything to eat or drink.

The hospital management might respond to the statement above with something like, "and correctly and justifiably so."

I will explain the concept of the Latin abbreviation NPO - or *nothing by mouth* for English language speakers - in detail in the following chapters.

If I were unfortunate enough to require a hospital stay again, I might elect to book a room at an expensive resort instead, and then just ask the front desk to call a doctor to my room to consult with me, should the need arise.

*****

Health insurance rates for working-age Americans have improved over the past decade. But not everyone with health insurance today has adequate financial protection.

About one-fourth of insured Americans are underinsured because they have significant coverage gaps or high out-of-pocket costs.

And all consumers are vulnerable to surprise medical bills, or balance bills for out-of-network care. These balance bills arise when insurance covers out-of-network care, but the provider bills the consumer for amounts beyond what the insurer pays and beyond cost-sharing, as well as in situations where out-of-network care is not normally covered but the selection of provider is outside the consumer's control.

Consumers are most likely to receive surprise medical bills from health providers outside their insurance plan's network after receiving emergency care or medical procedures at in-network facilities.

In the latter cases, for example, consumers may select a surgeon and facility in-network, but discover that other providers, such as an anesthesiologist or surgical assistant, are out of network.

These unexpected medical bills are a major concern for Americans. Some studies show nearly two-thirds of people surveyed say they are "very worried" or "somewhat worried" that they or a family member will receive a surprise bill.

In fact, these bills are the most-cited concern related to health care costs and other household expenses.

RUDIBESTER

*****

PART ONE

Personal Background

&

The Genesis
of Western Medicine

PROLOGUE

I was born and raised near Cape Town in South Africa, a coastal city near the southernmost tip of Africa.

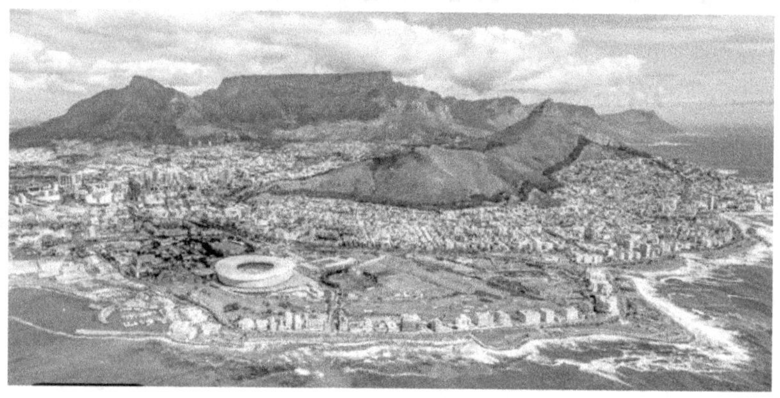

Many people who live in the "developed Western world", or in "First World countries" will often refer to South Africa as a *developing nation*.

As a child I was indoctrinated by a government-managed public education system, like most children. We therefore did not think of South Africa as a developing nation at all.

We were the best... at most anything and everything!

Our teachers taught us that when compared with many other countries, South Africa had few equals.

Relatively harmless state-sponsored propaganda included, for example, that South Africa had the greatest economy (in Africa anyway); one of the most powerful armies in the world; the best international rugby team; world-renowned agricultural crops of incomparable quality… fruits, wine, meats, and more.

The government informed us that we were able to be energy independent, and self-sufficient. After all, we had pioneered the manufacturing of gasoline from coal. The process - invented by a German chemist - had been perfected in South Africa by the state-owned energy company, SASOL.

Some of these *we are the best* categories above were hard to justify because we were never able to compare ourselves or compete head-to-head with many other countries, due to international isolation.

Informational media, products, etc. were government-censored and/or controlled. I did not know this at the time, only learning about it later.

*****

You might ask, "why are you sharing this information?"

The answer is because governments generally cannot be trusted, although they are often very effective marketers.

Mark Twain once said, "If you do not read the newspapers, you are uninformed. And if you do read the newspaper, you are misinformed."

Most information shared by government *experts* - especially when the topics are health related - is disinformation.

For example, when a bureaucrat says, *"eat this, not that"* or *"it is for your health"*, or *"if you take this vaccine, you will not get covid"*, etc.

...you are being misled.

Granted, the original intent might have been good.

Yet, poor advice propagated by government experts has historically delivered terrible outcomes e.g., an obesity epidemic, increases in chronic diseases, prescription drug dependencies, and even death.

At the time of my birth, smoking cigarettes was not even regarded as *unhealthy.*

It was only in 1964 that Luther L. Terry, Surgeon General of the U.S. Public Health Service, released the first health warning related to Smoking and Health.

The Centers for Disease and Control and Prevention, commonly known as the CDC, has scrubbed their website and archive. All historical promotional references related to *the promotion of cigarette smoking as being beneficial to people's health,* have been removed.

But today, their sister agency - the Food & Drug Administration, or FDA - is entrusted with the regulation, manufacture, import, packaging, labeling, advertising, promotion, sale, and distribution of cigarettes.

Therefore, when the FDA proclaims something as *safe and effective,* or good *for your health,* your *spidey senses** should immediately start tingling.

> ** Spidey sense generally refers to an extraordinary ability to sense imminent danger, thanks to the comic book hero, Spiderman.*

*****

Anyway, for the purposes of providing a little bit of South African history - as a developing nation - I thought to share a few interesting historical tidbits.

In the early eighties, I personally worked at a tabloid newspaper headquartered in Johannesburg - The Citizen - that had been created, funded, and controlled by the ruling National Party government.

It was a government propaganda mouthpiece, disguised as a source of objective news media. Of course, one cannot possibly know... what one does not know!

International sanctions against South Africa undermined domestic progress in the 80's, both from a general humanitarian point of view, and of course economically.

Competitively, we were lagging. But as a domiciled South African resident one would be none the wiser, thanks to ongoing government propaganda.

Sound familiar?

The examples shared above are probably not dissimilar to United States government agencies collaborating to convince honest, but often gullible, ordinary hard working Americans that Lee Harvey Oswald was a *single shooter*, and solely responsible for Pres. Kennedy's assassination.

****

Sanctions were imposed - on the South African people rather than only the government - by many global countries, as punishment for the ruling political party's abhorrent practice of legislated racial discrimination, called *apartheid*.

Apartheid, literally translated from Afrikaans, means separatism, or an ideology of *being separate.*

The problem with South Africa's institutionalized separation - at the time - was that it denied rights to anyone who was not classified as being of Caucasian descent.

Some South African pioneers and geniuses became world famous, despite sanctions.

At the time of writing, most people are probably familiar with Elon Musk?

Superstar inventor, visionary, entrepreneur, innovator... and wealthiest man in the world! Granted, he is a hero to some, and evil incarnate to others.

But many others had gone before, including people you might be familiar with.

Sporting heroes like Gary Player (who publicly denounced apartheid) successfully challenged and won several major global golfing titles.

South Africans also excelled in other fields, like medicine.

Prof. Christiaan Barnard was placed center stage in the world's spotlight when he performed the first ever human heart transplant on the 3rd of December 1967, at the Groote Schuur Hospital in Cape Town, South Africa.

South Africans also succeeded in international business.

Sir Ernest Oppenheimer, a Jewish-German émigré, founded the Anglo American Corporation (AAC) in 1917 in Johannesburg, South Africa. He had received financial backing from the American bank J.P. Morgan & Co. and raised £1 million from UK and US sources to start the gold mining company.

The company's name reflects the facts above.

The AAC became the majority stakeholder in the De Beers diamond company in 1926.

When Sir Ernest died in Johannesburg, he was succeeded as head of the company by his son Harry Fredrick Oppenheimer who became chairman of De Beers, the largest diamond company (or monopoly) in the world.

For many years, in South Africa, Harry Oppenheimer opposed apartheid, arguing that it hindered economic growth. Despite this, De Beers was often criticized for profiting from the system during the apartheid period.

By 1973, Anglo and De Beers accounted for 10 percent of South Africa's gross national product and 30 percent of the country's exports.

*****

When I was a kid growing up in South Africa, medical insurance - of any kind - did not exist.

For this primary reason, my personal experience, knowledge and/ or understanding of medical insurance schemes and how they operate was quite poor... until recently.

The history of *medical aid* in South Africa dates to the 80s, when some healthcare schemes were streamlined.

Once the benefits of subscribing to a medical aid scheme in the country became widely known, its popularity grew quickly. But the earliest types of medical aid schemes were merely hospital cash plans, rather than covers for payment of medical costs.

By the nineties, over 49 000 such policies had been sold.

The modern version of medical insurance had its origins in the fifties in the USA. It was then that cover payments were first introduced, paying for major medical procedures.

The original schemes in South Africa were only available to groups e.g., employers. Open medical aid enrollment options for individual members arrived much later.

By the early nineties several South African insurance companies were selling medical policies.

A *Dreaded Disease* policy had been introduced and became part of life insurance policies.

Medical aid, as available in South Africa today, is not medical insurance as we might know it or think of in the United States, but rather a plan that simply provides cover for day-to-day medical- and hospital costs.

This simply means that individuals pay a monthly contribution to the scheme, and in return the scheme pays service providers according to specified and agreed upon tariffs.

*****

For most of my early years, I cannot recall ever going to a doctor for a check-up, or simply because I felt ill.

My mother, who was my primary caregiver, died when I was twelve years old.

She treated all childhood illnesses with one, or a combination of: milk of magnesia, castor oil, black strap molasses, and mercurochrome (for cuts and scrapes).

Her healthcare philosophy was quite simple: if your tummy was fine and you had regular bowel movements at regular intervals... then you are also fine, and in good health.

There is some truth to this, but more about that later.

I do recall a doctor coming to our home when I was about five or six years old. This was a time when doctors still made house calls.

Dr. Martin had come to the house to vaccinate me. I have a vivid memory of this event.

One of my older brothers had generously taken his time to explain my upcoming experience in detail, so that I would be suitably prepared:

The doctor had various instruments of torture that he would be using to administer vaccines to various parts of my body. He also suitably prepared me for the good doctor's arrival by adding a warning about huge syringes with extraordinarily long, sharp needles.

The threat of my pending doom literally caused me to attempt to run away when Dr. Martin's car pulled up in the driveway! As a result of this experience, his name was etched into my memory, forever.

On one other occasion, when I was a few years older, I sustained a cut to my Achilles heel area from a rusty piece of metal in a children's playground.

The wound required stitches. This incident was my first experience of a hospital's emergency room.

After my mother's death at age twelve, I would never see another doctor (or dentist, nurse, etc.) for several years.

*****

As previously mentioned, my mother, who was also a single parent, had died when I was twelve years old.

I spent most of my teenage years living with my oldest brother and his wife and family. I am not sure we had a family doctor or some other primary healthcare provider, or service.

The next time I would personally see a doctor for a general check-up, was when I was about twenty years of age, and reporting for military service.

After having been declared fit, healthy, and deemed physically suitable and acceptable for active military duty, I was conscripted.

A few months later, I was working as an Ops Medic (EMS) in the army and saw doctors daily, but fortunately never as a patient.

Many people suggest that doctors and nurses make the worst patients. This observation might be true for me as well.

Later, after completing my military service, I became a sales representative for a leading drug company.

My professional work experience probably compounded my distrust of an assumed, ongoing *pursuit of good science* by pharmaceutical companies, in general.

For color, I will offer this amusing anecdote:

We sold an over-the-counter analgesic with a primary ingredient, paracetamol 500 mg.

It was used to treat minor aches and pains, and paracetamol also reduces fever.

We offered the same product - in tablet form - in several different colors. Mottled tablets offered extra strength.

But there was literally no difference between the different colored tablets, save for the packaging and marketing terms like XL, Extra Strength, 12-Hour, etc.

I was personally entrusted with a responsibility to deliver results that matched or exceeded my employer's aggressive sales targets for a portfolio of prescription drugs.

During the next decade - while still living in South Africa - I only visited consulting doctors occasionally. Obviously, this comment excludes my regular visits to doctors and hospitals for sales calls as a pharmaceutical representative, for professional business reasons.

My doctor's visits as a paying client were, for example, to support and accompany my wife during her doctor's visits related to her pregnancies (twice).

*****

CHAPTER 1: CARNEGIE, ROCKEFELLER & FLEXNER MEDICINE

E. Richard Brown's book - *Rockefeller medicine men: medicine and capitalism in America* - tells a hidden story of the financial, political, and institutional manipulation.

Brown describes a diverse and eclectic range of healing modalities available to the North American public that was summarily pared down to a singular style of medicine. The latter became the predominant medicine of the Western world, and a major force in global medical culture during the 20th century.

This change was brought about largely by the collaboration of the American Medical Association, the philanthropies of Andrew Carnegie and John D. Rockefeller, and the development of a revolutionary curriculum by the Johns Hopkins School of Medicine.

Brown documents the story of how a powerful professional elite gained virtual hegemony in the Western theater of healing by effectively taking control of the ethos and practice of Western medicine.

He describes how, in 1905, the American Medical Association's new Council on Medical Education funded by Carnegie and Rockefeller commenced serious activity.

They employed the services of Abraham Flexner who proceeded to visit and "assess" every single medical school in the US and Canada.

Within a short time of this development, medical schools all around the US began to collapse or consolidate.

By 1910, 30 schools had merged, and 21 had closed their doors. Of the 166 medical schools operating in 1904, 133 had survived by 1910, and 104 by 1915.

Fifteen years later, only 76 schools of medicine existed in the US. And they all followed the same curriculum.

Brown shows how both social and political processes were consciously manipulated by a medical elite acting in concert with immense corporate wealth to create a system of medicine that better served economic and hegemonic intentions than social or humanitarian needs.

- Extracted and edited from a Goodreads review

Brown's book was selected by scholars as being culturally important and is part of the knowledge base of civilization as we know it.

His work is in the public domain in the United States of America, and possibly other nations.

Within the United States, you may freely copy and distribute this work, as no entity (individual or corporate) has a copyright on the body of the work.

Scholars believe that this work is important enough to be preserved, reproduced, and made generally available to the public.

*****

CHAPTER 2: THE FLEXNER REPORT

The Flexner Report is listed as one of the most important publications in modern medicine.

It was a book-length *landmark* report of the medical education system in the United States and Canada, written by Abraham Flexner, and published in 1910 under the aegis of the Carnegie Foundation.

The Flexner Report is also referred to as *Carnegie Foundation Bulletin Number Four*.

Many aspects and policies of the present-day American medical profession stem from the Flexner Report.

It has been criticized for introducing policies that encouraged systemic racism, as illustrated below (pg. 180, Flexner Report).

A repercussion of the Flexner Report, resulting from the closure or consolidation of university training, was the closure of all but two "negro" medical schools.

CHAPTER XIV

THE MEDICAL EDUCATION OF THE NEGRO

THE medical care of the negro race will never be wholly left to negro physicians. Nevertheless, if the negro can be brought to feel a sharp responsibility for the physical integrity of his people, the outlook for their mental and moral improvement will be distinctly brightened. The practice of the negro doctor will be limited to his own race, which in its turn will be cared for better by good negro physicians than by poor white ones. But the physical well-being of the negro is not only of moment to the negro himself. Ten million of them live in close contact with sixty million whites. Not only does the negro himself suffer from hookworm and tuberculosis; he communicates them to his white neighbors, precisely as the ignorant and unfortunate white contaminates him. Self-protection not less than humanity offers weighty counsel in this matter; self-interest seconds philanthropy. The negro must be educated not only for his sake, but for ours. He is, as far as human eye can see, a permanent factor in the nation. He has his rights and due and value as an individual; but he has, besides, the tremendous importance that belongs to a potential source of infection and contagion.

The report called on American medical schools to enact higher admission and graduation standards, and to adhere strictly to the protocols of mainstream science in their teaching and research. It talked about the need to revamp and centralize medical institutions.

Many medical schools fell short of the standards required and advocated in the Flexner Report and nearly half of these schools merged or were closed outright.

Homeopathy, traditional osteopathy, eclectic medicine, and physiomedicalism (botanical therapies that had not been tested scientifically) were derided.

The Report also concluded that there were too many medical schools in the United States and that too many doctors were being trained.

Yet another outcome of the Report was the reversion of American universities to male-only admittance programs to accommodate a smaller admission pool (pg. 178, Flexner Report).

CHAPTER XIII

THE MEDICAL EDUCATION OF WOMEN

MEDICAL education is now, in the United States and Canada, open to women upon practically the same terms as men. If all institutions do not receive women, so many do, that no woman desiring an education in medicine is under any disability in finding a school to which she may gain admittance. Her choice is free and varied. She will find schools of every grade accessible: the Johns Hopkins, if she has an academic degree; Cornell, if she has three-fourths of one; Rush and the state universities, if she prefers the combined six years' course; Toronto on the basis of a high school education; Meridian, Mississippi, if she has had no definable education at all.

Universities had begun opening and expanding female admissions as part of women's and co-educational facilities only in the mid-to-latter part of the 19th century, but enrollment of women into medical schools declined (pgs. 178 & 179, Flexner Report)

Now that women are freely admitted to the medical profession, it is clear that they show a decreasing inclination to enter it. More schools in all sections are open to them; fewer attend and fewer graduate. True enough, medical schools generally have shrunk; but as the opportunities of women have increased, not decreased, and within a period during which entrance requirements have, so far as they are con-

MEDICAL EDUCATION OF WOMEN 179

cerned, not materially altered, their enrolment should have augmented, if there is any strong demand for women physicians or any strong ungratified desire on the part of women to enter the profession. One or the other of these conditions is lacking,—perhaps both.

When Flexner researched his report, "modern" medicine faced vigorous competition from several quarters, including osteopathic medicine, chiropractic medicine, electrotherapy, eclectic medicine, naturopathy, and homeopathy.

Flexner clearly doubted the scientific validity of all forms of medicine other than that based on scientific research, deeming any approach to medicine that did not advocate the use of treatments such as vaccines to prevent and cure illness as tantamount to quackery and charlatanism.

Medical schools that offered training in various disciplines including electromagnetic field therapy, phototherapy, eclectic medicine, physiomedicalism, naturopathy, and homeopathy, were told either to drop these courses from their curriculum or lose their accreditation and underwriting support.

A few schools resisted for a time, but eventually most complied with the Report or shut their doors.

*****

PART TWO

An Introduction to Canadian & American Healthcare Billing Scams
[& Related Shenanigans]

CHAPTER 3: OH CANADA!

My family and I arrived in Canada as permanent residents at the end of 1998.

Many people believe Canada has *free healthcare* and we therefore did not - initially anyway - consider purchasing any type of medical insurance.

When I landed my first job in Canada with a large company, my benefits package included a comprehensive family medical insurance plan. I was to be eligible for this benefit after three months of employment.

The cost of this insurance plan was split between my employer and myself, on a per pay basis, each paying half the cost. My pay stub included a line item, *Medical Insurance*.

This insurance plan was meant to cover all the expenses that Canada's *free healthcare* system did not cover, like medicine, eyeglasses, dental, etc.

My first experience using my new, paid-for dental insurance was, shall we say, *interesting*.

During that introductory visit to the dentist, he said, "We will help you to maximize your insurance". I was not sure exactly what this meant but I was too embarrassed to ask him.

I asked my neighbor who had originally introduced and recommended the dentist, to *translate* this for me.
She said that the dentist was simply offering to make sure we utilized the entire annual family dental insurance allocation, as per my employer's plan benefits, for my family and myself.

It meant, for example, that we would be able to enjoy regular checkups and cleanings, even if none were required.

I also quickly learned that a medical services provider - the dentist in my example above - would create a bill for a variety of services delivered, for each single visit.

For example: a dentist's bill might include a new set of x-rays (even if not required), professional cleaning done by an oral hygienist, a check-up by the dentist himself, sealants to help protect teeth from cavities, etc.

*****

I understand the basic business logic.

Previously, in South Africa, I had owned electronic retail stores. I trained my staff to ensure that customers would not leave our store with a single line item on their purchase receipt.

For example, when we sold a camera, the sales order receipt should include the camera, film, extra batteries, a cleaning kit... and perhaps even a carry bag and a tripod.

We - like most retailers - were able to generate more profit from add-on accessories, than from the sale of single cameras.

The simple sales strategy of trying to generate bills with multiple line items results in increases to both revenue and profitability.

And, as shared above, I had previously worked for one of the largest pharmaceutical companies on the planet for a few years. I managed sales for a large region. As such, I had a reasonably good idea of my management responsibilities and objectives, or sales quotas.

The primary business objective of the entire healthcare, medical, and pharmaceutical industries, and their affiliates... is profit generation.

Pharmaceutical corporations need to lock people into repeat prescriptions for various ailments, rather than offer a drug that cures *something*.

If they offered a cure, most of their ongoing, recurring, profitable, net new revenue would be gone!

Even doctors asking patients to return for example, a month after an initial appointment, allows them to bill another consult, rather than requesting your return for the primary purpose of checking in on your health status.

The generalizations above exclude healthcare workers who really care about their clients, and there are many who do.

Caring practitioners are often easily identified by their follow-up actions. For example, they might contact a client a few days after an initial visit and/or medical procedure, just to find out if the client is doing alright.

After all, following up to ensure that everything is *okay* can be accomplished by making a simple telephone call or sending an email, most of the time.

*****

Thus, when I presented for my regular 6-monthly teeth cleaning appointment - a 40-minute service that was realistically worth less than $100 in time and materials - the dentist presented me with a total bill for e.g., $900.

I would then pay 20% - or $180 out of pocket - and the insurance company would take care of the outstanding balance, albeit at their negotiated, predetermined, discounted rates for the services delivered.

However, even though I could not be certain, I assumed that there was no way the insurance company would fork out their share of the bill - $720 - for relatively simple and arguably unnecessary services, as described above... from the goodness of their heart!

If I were to be generous and suggest that my insurance company had settled the *remaining, outstanding balance* for e.g., $200, the dentist still effectively generated nearly $400 worth of revenue for a service that started off as a simple, regular teeth-cleaning procedure, worth $100.

But I learned that this was simply how the great healthcare billing scam, for insured patients, worked.

*****

CHAPTER 4: THE LAND OF THE BRAVE AND THE FREE

We arrived in Florham Park, New Jersey, from Toronto as new, permanent U.S. residents mid-2008.

It was early summer. Right at the start of the greatest financial and economic collapse since the Great Depression of 1929.

At the time, I was employed as a senior executive for a Canadian financial services company.

Some job-related benefits I immediately enjoyed because of our migration to the U.S. - like lower income taxes - were partially offset by higher costs on payroll deductions for line items like medical insurance.

Regardless, I was suddenly flush with additional monthly disposable income, more so than before.

The above was true because the embedded cost of Canada's supposedly *free healthcare system* was obvious to observe in my suddenly much larger take-home after-tax pay, from the very first month!

In Canada my personal tax rate was above 50%.

This rate was a combination of federal, provincial, and sales taxes. The latter, at the time, was 15% on pretty much anything we purchased except fresh food, children's clothing, and a few other exempt items.

In New Jersey the local state income- and sales taxes, added together, were already less than Toronto's 15% sales tax.

Therefore, for starters, I was saving at least the additional amount that had previously been deducted from my gross pay for Ontario's provincial tax, proverbially speaking. And, ironically, New Jersey would be considered *a high tax state* by many Americans!

But furthermore, literally everything was *cheaper* than in Canada. The cost of gasoline was about half. Basic groceries were probably 20-30% less expensive. Technology (cable, cell phone, internet, etc.) costs were also about half of what I had been paying in Canada.

But at that time, I had not yet experienced the greatest American con ever... the healthcare billing scam!

CHAPTER 5:
DERMATOLOGY,
LESSON ONE

In 2010, after having lived in the United States for about two years, I decided to go and see a dermatologist.

There was a dermatology practice conveniently located directly across the street from our house, so I decided to visit that doctor's practice.

I was employed full time at the time. My employer's benefits package included good medical insurance.

I checked to see whether specialist doctor visits would be covered, and yes, it was.

A few years ago, while we were living in Canada, our family practitioner had referred me to a dermatologist for seborrheic keratosis removal.

It took nearly four months before I was able to see the dermatologist in Toronto. But remember, in Canada healthcare is *free* and managed by the government, and therefore long waiting times are common. And anyway, in my case, there had been no urgency.

My family doctor had informed me that the lesions were basically harmless. The procedure to remove the lesions was simple and more cosmetic than medically required.

A seborrheic keratosis is a common non cancerous, or benign skin growth. People tend to get more of them as they get older.

The lesions are usually small, and brown, black, or light tan in appearance. The growths look waxy or scaly and are often slightly raised. They appear gradually, usually on the face, neck, chest, or back.

For most people, in general, seborrheic keratoses are harmless, and not contagious.

They do not require treatment. A person may decide to have them removed if they become irritated by clothing or if you do not like how they look, especially if they were present and visible on your face.

Removal can be achieved by freezing the growth.

Freezing a lesion with liquid nitrogen (cryotherapy) is an effective, simple, and inexpensive way to remove a seborrheic keratosis. This is what I had experienced before, in Canada.

This procedure took only a few seconds, although the doctor had spent several minutes with me... mostly for billing purposes, I assume.

This time, now a few years later, I would experience *the same procedure* in the United States as a patient insured by a private company, as opposed to my costs being covered by a government's public healthcare system.

On the day of my visit the front office staff presented me with many forms to complete, as is common for new patients.

They captured my personal information, insurer's details, and required my sign-off related to liability waivers, privacy laws, etc.

Standard administrivia.

Eventually, I was taken into a consulting room where I would see the doctor.

I shared the information above, as related to my previous experience in Canada, and - using an index finger – pointed out some new lesions on my face. I did this because I could feel the keratoses, which were not easily visible to an observer.

The doctor asked me to remove my clothing so that he could examine the skin on other parts of my body.

Clothed only in my underwear for a consultation related to keratosis on my face, was very different from my experience in Canada, where I had merely been seated on a chair facing the doctor.

The American doctor then proceeded to examine my entire body - from my scalp to my feet - for signs of any other dermatologically related conditions that might require his attention and/or treatment.

I was quite impressed!

They had not examined me to this extent in Canada.

My new, very efficient American doctor advised me that he would do some scraping - called curettage - shaving the skin's surface in some areas.

First, he numbed the few areas under investigation, and then used a scalpel blade to remove a growth.

When he had finished the cryotherapy, complete physical examination, and curettage, I got dressed again.

During this time and for a few minutes afterwards, we chatted, and he educated me about skincare in general, the use of sunscreen, he inquired about my diet and lifestyle, and covered other topics related to maintaining a good, healthy skin.

I left the consulting room and on my way past reception I inquired about payment. They said that they would bill the insurance company directly and send me an invoice for my co-pay portion.

For people not familiar with co-pay, that is the portion of the bill that I would personally be responsible for.

A common copay percentage is twenty percent.

The above means that a patient might be required to pay the first twenty percent of the doctor's invoice, and then the insurance company would accept responsibility for the remaining balance.

The example above does not imply that the insurance company would pay eighty percent of the invoice. Insurers have preset rates or arrangements with providers, affording them discounted rates.

I received the doctor's invoice a few days later in the mail.

The total amount billed was $2,800. My co-pay for the consultation and examination was 20% of the bill, and therefore $560 out of pocket.

I was somewhat stunned by the total cost of the entire adventure. But being none the wiser at the time, I sent the doctor's office a payment for *my portion*, and that was the end of that.

Next time I would know …and do better!

*****

CAUTION & WARNING!

THIS SECTION SHOULD NOT BE VIEWED AS MEDICAL ADVICE. I ENCOURAGE CRITICAL THOUGHT COMPLEMENTED BY RESEARCH, RATHER THAN LEMMING-LIKE COMPLIANCE TO QUESTIONABLE MANDATES.

BASICALLY, YOU SHOULD QUESTION EVERYTHING!

CHAPTER 6: DERMATOLOGY, LESSON TWO

About eight years went by before I saw a dermatologist again.

Sometime during 2018, I had developed a small lesion on the upper side of my right hand.

In size, it was about half the diameter of a penny. Initially I thought that I had damaged my skin somehow by scraping it on a rough surface, and that the small wound would eventually become a scar and heal naturally.

I am specifically mentioning the upper side of my hand because that would be a body part most exposed to the sun.

I had lived in South Africa for thirty six years. Cars are all right-hand-drive. That is also why I mentioned my right hand above.

Three and a half decades of blisteringly hot African sunshine, no use of sunscreen ever, and even having exposure to the sun while driving right-handed with the sun shining through the window... probably combine to create a great environment for nurturing a basal cell carcinoma.

Basal cell carcinoma is a type of skin cancer that most often develops on areas of skin exposed to the sun, such as the face.

For my second planned visit to a US dermatologist, I was a little wiser than the previous time.

I called a couple of dermatologists' consulting rooms.

I said I did not have medical insurance and asked how much a consultation would be if I paid them in cash.

Several dermatologist practices said they would not accept patients without insurance. That would be their right, so I thanked them, and simply called the next one.

Eventually, I found a dermatologist located near my office, who charged a base, cash fee of $175 for a consultation.

As it was, at that time I did have medical insurance. But my annual deductible was $8,000.

This means that for whatever medical expenses I incurred, I would be liable to pay *the first $8,000*.

After reaching that cap, the insurance company would start contributing to my medical expenses according to their plan documents that outline coverage limits, eligible services, etc.

In the context of my high deductible, sharing that I did not have medical insurance was partly true, and partly deceitful.

Generally, a mostly healthy person might not reach the annual deductible of $8,000 …and therefore end up paying for all medical expenses out-of-pocket anyway.

I therefore visited the doctor as *a cash patient*.

She examined the lesion on my hand. She scraped or shaved a sample, to send to a lab.

I mentioned a couple of new keratoses spots on my face. She froze these for me at no additional cost. She also examined my back and arms as part of her investigation of my skin.

A few days after this appointment, her assistant called my office to let me know the sample they had scraped from my hand had returned a positive basal carcinoma diagnosis.

I asked about next steps. She said the doctor would need to do Mohs surgery to remove the carcinoma.

I inquired about what the outcome would be if we did nothing, given that it was so small and that the scrape had nearly removed all of it anyway.

She said it was unlikely to spread and added that it certainly was not life threatening.

But she asked, "Why would you want to live with a basal cell carcinoma on any part of your body?"

Good question!

I said that I would think about it and get back to them.

*****

Then I started my investigation, doing research on the Internet.

I am referring to reading medical research reports and peer reviewed case studies - as is my disposition - rather than visiting chat rooms on social media where people aimlessly gossip and opine about random topics that they are often completely unfamiliar with.

I learned that the average patient cost of Mohs surgery was about $2,575. The price for cash patients - people with no insurance - could be as high as $12,000.

Of course, Mohs surgery costs vary widely, depending on the specifics of the procedure and a few other key factors, like the location of the lesion.

My basal cell carcinoma, being small and on my hand, would be at the lower end of any price range.

Larger lesions e.g., on a patient's face, would probably be at the higher end of any price range, for obvious reasons.

*****

I learned about Imiquimod cream.

Imiquimod is not an immunosuppressant.

It is, in fact: *"an immunomodulator that acts as a toll-like receptor-7 agonist and activates macrophages and other immune cells. It promotes interferon-alpha, tumor necrosis factor-alpha, and other cytokines to increase TH1-type immunity."*

-   Urosevic & Dummer, 2004

A four-week (12 sachet) treatment of 5% Imiquimod, 250mg strength, cost about $36.00 at the time of writing.

But what exactly is Imiquimod?

In the United States, this topical cream requires a prescription from a doctor, and it is most used to treat external genital warts (in people over the age of 12).

Imiquimod can be used to fight the warts, but it does not cure the underlying virus that causes the warts.

Patients apply Imiquimod at night and it encourages their immune cells to attack the warts.

Wonderful stuff!

But how does Imiquimod work?

By stimulating a person's immune system to help identify abnormal cells. This produces inflammation and encourages the immune system to combat genital warts.

And what can Imiquimod be used for?

Well, it works by helping your immune system to identify abnormal cells. Therefore, Imiquimod can be used for genital warts, actinic keratosis, and basal cell carcinoma (an early form of skin cancer).

The primary purpose for sharing this information is to illustrate that it is always useful to inquire about alternative treatments, options that might be available, off-label use of older medicines that are generally safe and might be useful for other afflictions.

By the way, one would be ill advised trying to use Google to diagnose medical conditions. One can, however, use the Internet to become better informed. And then, one would be well advised to ask a medical professional to professionally and expertly diagnose and/or confirm any affliction.

By being more knowledgeable, you can have intelligent conversations with your medical provider, and perhaps even offer assistance and insight… but that is all.

*****

Based on my research, the location of my basal cell carcinoma, and the small size of the lesion, I decided to attempt self-treatment with Imiquimod cream.

It worked, cleared up the lesion, although I ended up needing two treatments i.e., using it for eight weeks.

Although Imiquimod requires a prescription in the United States, it is sold over the counter ("OTC") in many countries.

Imiquimod side effects - as per the package insert - includes mainly skin-related issues; like redness, swelling, a rash, burning, flaking, etc.

I experienced none of the above.

My total cost for the treatment of my basal cell carcinoma was about $100 plus several hours of my time, doing research.

For more than four years - at the time of writing - the skin on my hand appears to be healthy. I have no visible scarring, nor any other damage.

*****

PART THREE

The Great American Healthcare Billing Scam

CHAPTER 7: THEY KNOW NOTHING!

Now, before you chastise me for daring to accuse our great medical practitioners of knowing nothing, allow me to explain what I mean by nothing.

As **body mechanics** they know how to do certain things quite well, for example, tending to a fractured limb or stitching a wound. People have been doing this for centuries, and today we have modernized versions of these skills that could be described as *fine art*, practiced by highly specialized people.

Just recently, two of our clients had knee and hip replacement surgeries, respectively. Both are doing exceptionally well, moving freely and without any pain, and probably in better condition today, than previously.

As **technology experts** they are well trained to know and understand how modern diagnostic machines work, what these machines can or cannot do, the usefulness of the equipment in certain circumstances, etc. Here I am referring to X-ray, CAT, MRI, EKG, etc. to diagnose various medical conditions. Without the machine, the technology experts are often, arguably, completely useless.

As **drug pushers** - in a legal sense - the chemical experts have a cure for every disease. Or so it would seem.

One ER doctor proudly told me that they have a more potent drug for any of my ailments, than the ailment itself. In simple terms... If you were experiencing level-8 pain, they have a level-9 analgesic to inject into you, and so on.

As a general rule, emergency room ("ER") or Emergency Medical Services ("EMS") technicians are the most highly skilled professional human body mechanics and fixer-uppers.

These guys often work under enormous pressure, are required to make life-and-death decisions quickly, and face uncertainty every time medical emergencies present.

If you are fortunate to live near an ER nurse, you have won the jackpot and you might never require medical attention from anyone else.

Excluding the EMS pros, generally speaking, the other medical professionals mentioned above, know nothing!

Healthcare, by definition, should be about **health**, and **care**.

Although there are many exceptions to my "They know Nothing" accusation - like my examples of ER and EMS technicians above - most healthcare workers do not care much about your health.

But they do care about money!

*****

Day One

Saturday, March 26th, 2022.

I woke up at 4:36 AM.

The reason for the early wakeup was severe abdominal pain, unlike anything I had ever experienced before.

I got up, walked around a bit, had a few sips of water, and thought the pain would subside or dissipate after a while.

But alas, it was not to be.

A few hours later I showered and got dressed, expecting a regular day.

I prepared a light breakfast. One slice of toast with marmalade and a cup of coffee.

Later that morning, I drove to our charitable gift shop - where I usually spend my Saturdays - and expected my condition to improve as the day went by.

Just before noon I left the shop and walked to a nearby walk-in clinic. These clinics are popular, especially for people who are under-insured, or who have no insurance.

I paid a $125 cash fee on arrival, for a doctor's consultation.

*****

In general, walk-in clinics offer uninsured, cash payers reduced prices, and resist upselling uninsured patients, for obvious reasons.

Their healthcare practitioners also tend to see patients faster than a traditional doctor's room, probably because they have more staff, for example, when compared with a single family practitioner's office.

I was no longer employed by a large corporation, with a benefits package that included medical insurance.

In good faith, I had purchased an Affordable Care Act insurance policy every year since retiring from my professional career, in 2014.

The Affordable Care Act - formally known as the Patient Protection and Affordable Care Act of 2010 - is better known as, or commonly referred to, as *Obamacare*.

My *Obamacare* plan had an $8,700 deductible (the amount I would need to expend before the insurance would pay for anything).

I am comfortable with such a high deductible for these few reasons: my personal financial situation was/is sound, and I am in generally good health. The latter is due to good genes (I assume), daily exercise, a good diet, etc.

Regrettably, my comments directly above do not apply to the average American enrolled into an *Obamacare* medical insurance plan.

Most Americans are not *financially healthy*.

More importantly, they are not generally in good physical health. Many Americans do not exercise regularly, and collectively we consume more prepackaged, processed, high-fat foods, than most people on earth.

*****

A nurse practitioner at the walk-in clinic saw me in her examination room at around noon.

I shared information about my early morning adventures and added that the pain had now become severe enough for me to present at her clinic.

My mere presence at the clinic, I added, was an extraordinary event for me because I would usually avoid going to any medical facilities, whenever possible.

She inquired about my general health, diet, and more specifically about the dinner I had eaten the previous evening.

She asked me to lay down on an examination bed and pushed and prodded around my abdomen. Usually, at this time, a healthcare practitioner would start by eliminating more obvious conditions like an inflamed appendix, for example.

Due to her inability to identify a specific reason for my pain, she suggested that we take an abdominal x-ray.

"This would be an additional $122", she added.

I agreed.

A front office desk clerk was summoned.

She arrived with a portable, handheld card payment machine in hand - the kind they use at restaurants - and charged my debit card.

A staff member then escorted me to the x-ray room.

The x-ray took a few minutes. The nurse practitioner who had consulted with me earlier said that she would send it to the doctor, and that they would call later with the results.

To date, at the time of writing a few months later, I still do not know the results of that x-ray.

In their defense, they did call my mobile phone number a few days after my visit and left a voicemail inquiring about my health.

*****

The nurse practitioner diagnosed my condition as food poisoning. She gave me a prescription for two drugs: one for nausea and the other for gastric reflux.

Then, she sent me on my way, and I left, prescription in hand.

Back at the charitable gift shop, now around 1:30 PM, I informed our team that I was not feeling well.

I went home.

*****

Just after 3 PM I called my wife.

I told her that I was now experiencing excruciating abdominal pain, and that I had started vomiting. In no condition to drive, I told her that I would call 911 and ask the ambulance to take me to the nearest emergency room.

My wife said she could be home in minutes and asked me to wait for her to get home, so that she could take me to the ER.

I declined. I felt that I needed medical care immediately and without any unnecessary delay.

An ambulance arrived within 10 minutes of my call.

Inside the ambulance, the medic asked for my insurance information. I had remembered to take my medical insurance ID card with me before they picked me up.

They then proceeded to prepare me for the ER drop-off.

For context, American healthcare service providers always first ask for a patient's medical insurance information before attending to the patient, unless he or she is totally incapacitated and unable to converse.

The EMS medic, a first responder quite efficient and adept at attending to diverse medical emergency situations, readied me for a drip, checked my vitals, and chatted with me all the way to the ER.

Patients in severe pain typically appreciate the calm confidence and ongoing, reassuring communication of a trained professional attending to them.

A few minutes later they wheeled me into the emergency room of a medical center - located nearest to my home where they had picked me up - and handed me over to the hospital's ER team.

This point above is important. I had not selected the emergency room, or hospital.

The ambulance took me to the ER facility located closest to my home because, for them, time is always of essence and their job is to take a patient to the nearest critical care facility.

I was blissfully unaware that medical insurance companies have out-of-network hospitals. If a facility is out of their network, the insurance company will refuse to pay for *anything*.

*****

In this - my first lesson about the Great American Healthcare Billing Scam - I learned that before an ambulance picks up a patient, the patient first needs to call his or her insurance company to ask where - i.e., to which ER or hospital - they should be taken.

People should have confidence in the knowledge that if they need emergency care, they should be able to go to the nearest emergency room, and that their insurance will cover whatever transpires in relation to their health and wellbeing, from that moment on.

Note: contrary to negative comments by many critics, not everything about Obamacare is bad, a failure or terrible.

Many people have benefitted from this divisive piece of legislation that Congress passed, despite all the animosity and infighting between opposing politicians.

One good feature of *Obamacare* is that it requires all plans to cover emergency services.

Insurers cannot charge their clients more for going to an out-of-network hospital or health care provider's emergency room. The insurer also cannot require patients to get pre-authorization before receiving ER service.

However, people should be aware of these issues:

1. An "emergency" is usually a situation that is life-threatening, or one that could result in the loss of a limb in the absence of immediate medical attention.
2. Obamacare requires insurers to cover emergency services at the same price, whether a hospital is in or out of network.
3. Even if your insurance covers it, an emergency room visit can still leave you with thousands of dollars in unexpected medical bills.
4. Urgent care centers can be a cheaper and faster option for situations that are not life-threatening.

I also learned a second lesson about the Great American Healthcare Billing Scam from my experience: emergency physicians are often independent contractors.

They do not work primarily for that hospital, and so they could very well be out-of-network health care providers for you, even if the hospital is in your insurer's network.

In the end, you will pay according to the negotiated rates between your insurance and the ER.

You will also pay any fees that your insurance will not cover because you went to a hospital, ER, or doctor who is out of network.

Other costs are also added to your bill, like the cost of an ambulance if you took one to the hospital but your insurer determines that you had other, cheaper transportation options.

*****

The main function of an emergency room is usually to treat life-threatening illnesses and injuries.

They have advanced diagnostic equipment and access to more types of medicine than a primary care doctor might have.

Note that they will use *all* their diagnostic machines and bill you for their use of those machines, as appropriate.

*****

After my arrival, the ER team attached electrodes to my chest to perform an EKG, or ECG. These are acronyms for the word *electrocardiography*.

On one hand, one might argue that an EKG was not necessary. On the other hand, the ER's specialist medical team was seeking to eliminate a potential heart problem as a cause for the patient's yet undiagnosed pain.

An EKG produces an electrocardiogram. This is a recording of the heart's electrical activity.

Medical staff will perform a basic test of a patient's vital signs. These include checking the patient's body temperature, pulse rate, respiration rate (or rate of breathing) and blood pressure. The EKG complements the check of vital signs.

Each of these procedures carries its own price tag.

As explained above, some of these tasks will be performed by independent contractors who might be out-of-network, even if the hospital or ER happens to be in-network for your insurance company.

*****

A doctor on call came to see me. I explained my situation and how I came about being at the ER.

Our conversation was interesting, to say the least. It went something like this:

Doctor: What did you have to eat last night?

Me: I had sausage, rice, avocado, and a slice of naan.

Doctor: Was it take-out rice?

Me: No, I made it myself.

Doctor: Freshly cooked?

Me: No, I made it a few days ago and put it in the freezer. I heated it up in the microwave before I ate it.

Doctor: That is a bad idea. It was the rice. You should not do that. Only eat it freshly cooked, straight out of the pot.

Me: Oh, I did not know that. I have been cooking rice, freezing it, and eating it later for years!

Doctor: It was the rice. Rice contains bacteria that causes food poisoning. Your food poisoning is quite severe.

Me: Oh, thank you, that is good to know.

He instructed the duty nurse to give me a shot of morphine for my abdominal pain.

*****

They drew blood for lab tests and requested a urine sample.

After being stabilized (primarily for pain), they proceeded to send me for some diagnostic tests.

These included magnetic resonance imaging (MRI). This diagnostic medical imaging technique uses a magnetic field and computer-generated radio waves to create detailed images of the organs and tissues in your body.

The next test was a computed tomography (CT or CAT) scan.

For the diagnostic machine nerds, a CAT scan allows doctors to see inside your body. It uses a combination of X-rays and a computer to create pictures of your organs, bones, and other tissues. It shows more detail than a regular X-ray.

When the tests had all been completed, I spent another few hours lying on the ER hospital gurney, waiting for whatever might happen next.

At this stage, I had been in the emergency room for several hours, and it was close to midnight.

Eventually the doctor returned. He chatted with me for a few minutes about which foods I should eat, foods to avoid, and clear energy drinks I could consume for the next couple of days until I recovered.

I said that if my condition were severe food poisoning, I would like to go home.

He agreed, and gave me a prescription for two drugs, not the same, but like the ones that had been prescribed for me earlier that day by the nurse practitioner at the walk-in clinic: one for nausea and the other for gastric reflux:

Protonix 40 mg oral enteric coated tablet

Date Started On: Mar 26, 2022

Zofran 8 mg oral tablet Learn more

Date Started On: Mar 26, 2022

I did not sleep much that night.

In between bouts of abdominal pain and cramping, I also had to get up a few times during the night because I kept feeling nauseous, even though I had not eaten for a day.

Day Two

Sunday, March 27th, 2022

The following morning my wife went to a drugstore nearby and filled the prescription for me.

My chosen diet was Gatorade.

But every time I drank Gatorade, I would vomit. And every time after vomiting, I would drink more Gatorade.

I figured that if I just kept drinking a sports-beverage, I would at least be getting some hydration. And after all, this product was intended to help athletes refuel, recover, and perform.

Day Three

Monday, March 28th, 2022.

I decided that 2-3 days would be required to *get this bug out of my system.*

I spent the day lounging around at home, reading, drinking sports drinks, vomiting occasionally, and napping from time to time.

I tried to eat some simple foods, like a bowl of soup that included a slice of bread broken into bits, but I only managed to keep it down for a few minutes.

Anyway, it was not that bad. I had some over the counter painkillers on hand along with the medication that had been prescribed for me.

However, my prescription medication was really of no use.

For one, I did not feel nauseous before vomiting, and secondly, hardly experienced gastric reflux that somehow needed to be controlled. But I took the medication anyway as prescribed, despite its inefficacy.

Day Four

Tuesday March 29th, 2022.

I was not getting better.

I had been suffering abdominal pain for several days.

I had not had a bowel movement for more than three days. I had not eaten any solid food for three days. My diet of sports drinks was not working as planned.

I was losing weight, getting weaker by the day, with no obvious sense of recovery.

I booked an in-home mobile IV therapy service for the next day.

Their website advertised a *Mobile & In-home IV Therapy for Food Poisoning* that is a carefully formulated blend of vitamins, fluids, medications, and electrolytes to mitigate any symptoms of food poisoning.

This Food Poisoning IV Drip also helps to shorten sickness time and promotes recovery. It helped to target food poisoning, fatigue, stomach aches, and low energy levels.

The concoction they would administer intravenously included the usual drip of fluids, anti-nausea medication, Pepcid, Glutathione, Zinc, NSAID, B-Complex Vitamins, Vitamin B12, and Vitamin C.

Day Five

Wednesday, March 30th, 2022.

The day after another sleepless night.

I bided my time laying around. I did some more reading. I drank many sports drinks, followed by as many trips to the bathroom. If I was not able to make it to the bathroom on time, a plastic bucket conveniently placed next to my bed sufficed.

The nurse from the IV therapy company arrived that afternoon at around 2 PM.

I paid $275 cash for the treatment.

Her procedure took about an hour.

I did not experience any observable benefit or change to my condition from the IV therapy. This often happens when one adopts an incorrect solution to a poorly diagnosed problem, I would guess.

I decided that I really needed to *get this bug out of my system*, so I spent the entire night in the bathroom… dividing my time between severe bouts of random vomiting and feeling sorry for myself, while sitting on the bathroom floor.

By now, I was even avoiding having sports drinks, because it just caused me to vomit immediately afterwards.

My sweet wife, the ultimate warrior, spent that same night in our spare room, not sleeping at all, and suffering with me, albeit in silence!

Day Six

Thursday March 31st, 2022.

"Houston, we have a problem!"

We were already closing in on a week since my early-morning awakening the previous Saturday.

By now, my food poisoning from a week prior should have been gone, but I was not getting better. Instead, I was progressively getting worse.

It was not so much that the pain had intensified. My abdominal pain was ever-present, but tolerable. The constant vomiting was symptomatic of my worsening condition, especially considering that I had now stopped eating and drinking entirely.

By that evening, I realized that I was experiencing a serious health issue.

My wife helped me into the car, and I returned to the same ER where that ambulance had taken me nearly a week prior.

A different ER doctor came to see me. He conducted the same diagnostic tests as I had described above in Day One.

However, this time he confidently said that I have a Small Bowel Obstruction. He would admit me to the adjoining hospital.

I waited in the ER for many hours until a room was ready and available for me. In the early morning hours of April 1st, they wheeled my ER gurney into a hospital room.

Day Seven

Friday, April Fool's Day, 2022

This date above was the start of my first experience as an in-patient *victim*.

I chose the naming convention above - rather than referring to myself as a patient - because the *victims* of the Great American Healthcare Billing Scam are figuratively viewed as automated banking machines that generate nearly unlimited amounts of revenue for the large corporations that own medical centers and hospitals.

To this end, April Fool's Day is quite apt as a descriptive date related to my introduction into the great scam.

*****

Regardless of how well your hospital treated your illness or injury, sadly, the healthcare system's billing structure is confusing and can often end up with the patient getting screwed over.

The reality is, healthcare is expensive, and hospitals and insurance companies are multi-million-dollar businesses that surround themselves with highly skilled people to protect their interests, and bottom line.

Meanwhile, individual patients can get stuck with exorbitant medical bills, making it difficult to carry on with normal life.

*****

All the diagnostic tests I described earlier, above, were repeated.

As a bonus, that Friday morning the duty nurse inserted a nasogastric (NG) tube. This medical intubation process involves the insertion of a plastic tube through the nose, down through the esophagus, and into the stomach.

The *other end* of the NG tube was attached to a small bedside plastic tank, which was - in turn - attached to a small pump i.e., a mechanical medical drainage system.

NG tubes enable doctors to feed and provide certain medications to people temporarily unable to swallow anything.

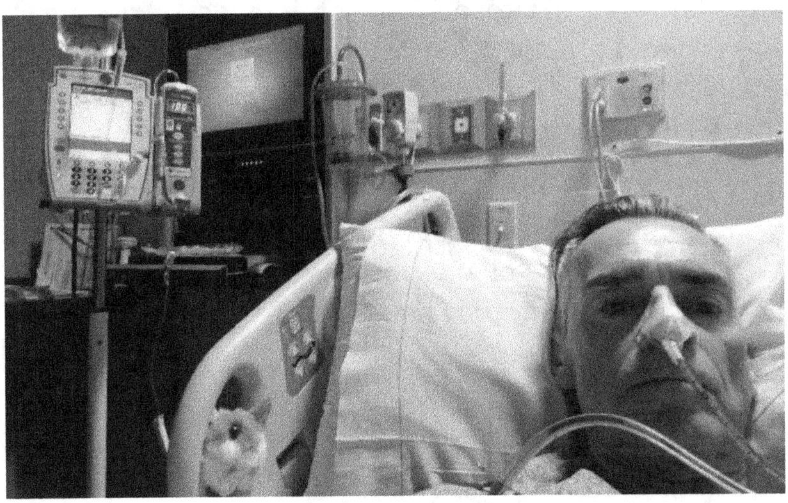

But it is also a common way to treat a small bowel obstruction (SBO), or intestinal blockage, used to remove substances from the stomach. This latter description was applicable in my instance.

The tube removes fluids and gas and helps to relieve pain and pressure. Patients are not given anything to eat or drink.

Most bowel obstructions are partial blockages that get better on their own over the course of a few days.

An NG tube generally helps the bowel to become unblocked when fluids and gas are mechanically removed.

****

Additional in-patient services include a nurse checking in every hour or so during daylight hours, and about every few hours during the night.

The standard care protocols do not include retrieving status updates from the patient. On the contrary, the nurses simply arrive and do their assigned tasks, nearly disregarding the patient's well being entirely.

For clarity, the statement above implies the following: If a nurse following a standard protocol and maintenance schedule needs to change a drip, take a blood sample, check vital signs, etc., they will do exactly whatever they have been instructed to do… and no more.

I commented above, "Most bowel obstructions are partial blockages that get better on their own."

I did not know this. The gastric surgeon, subcontracted to the hospital, told me this when he consulted with me in my hospital room.

He said, "SBO usually clears by itself in about 3-4 days. If yours has not done so by next Monday, we will have to operate, to see what is going on. That would not be desirable, and we would like to avoid that."

"Me too", I responded.

Day Eight

Saturday, April 2nd, 2022.

My older son flew in from Canada. He had been informed that his dad was ill, in hospital as an in-patient.

To help cheer me up, he hand-delivered a letter to me, from his son, my grandson, who was seven years old.

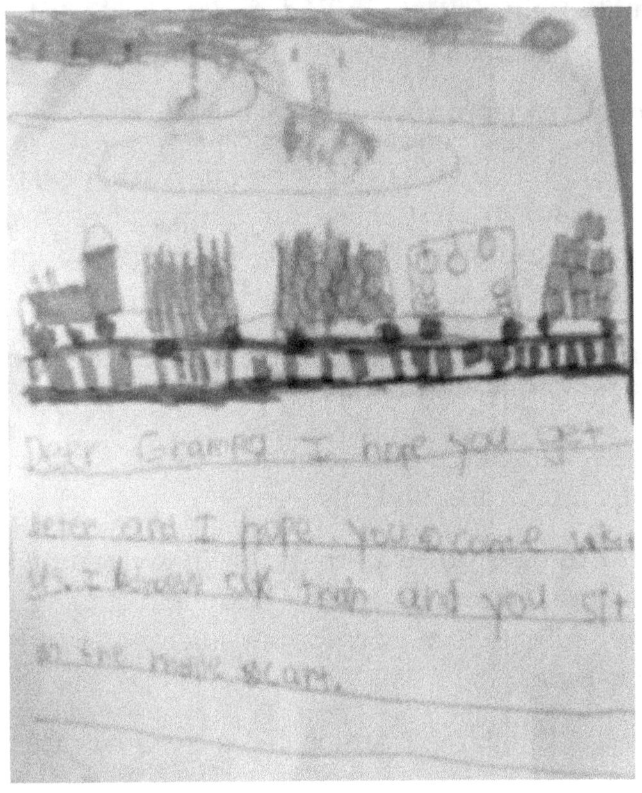

*****

Via the Internet I learned that a High Grade Small Bowel Obstruction leads to a fatality, 24% of the time.

Viewed optimistically then, I had a chance to see my son - whom I had not visited for two years due to Canadian Covid-19 lockdowns - because of my hospitalization.

Without even searching too much, one can always find a proverbial silver lining behind every cloud!

*****

Meanwhile, I was lying in my hospital bed, bored and unknowingly being *slowly milked financially* by the hospital's billing system, as the nurses did their regular rounds.

Their standard care protocol requires regular visits.

These in-room nurse visits might be interpreted as, figuratively speaking, an 80/20 split: 80% for billing purposes, 20% for patient care. An example of the Pareto principle, masquerading as patient care.

While lying in hospital, I read a book: *The Real Anthony Fauci* by Robert F. Kennedy, Jr.

It offers a detailed, documented history of corruption, bureaucratic ineptitude, and misdeeds.

As the name implies, the lead character in Kennedy's book about healthcare "pandemics", dangerous and ineffective vaccines, and other related misdeeds by corrupt bureaucrats... is the infamous Dr. Anthony Fauci.

It is a good, but tough read. Almost like a criminal case transcript.

The book documents Fauci's disastrous and borderline criminal career, spanning more than four decades.

Kennedy includes several, easily verifiable references to Fauci's AIDS/HIV campaign, a few pandemics along the way, and culminating with his latest efforts... the gain-of-function research that gave birth to the most recent global (2019) coronavirus pandemic.

To be clear, Fauci did not create the virus, he merely funded it.

He is also not directly responsible for killing people... he merely ignored any treatment protocols not recommended by his bureaucratic peers, big pharma cohorts, and supportive people of dubious medical standing, like Bill Gates.

Fauci worked tirelessly to silence any counterpoint to his official, preferred narrative. He even had the audacity to suggest that people who questioned him were, in fact, "questioning science".

Fauci's unbridled hubris appears to have no equal, save perhaps for that same trait generally displayed by career politicians.

But I digress.

*****

Day Nine

Sunday, April 3rd, 2022.

I learned that my sophisticated, automatic, motorized hospital bed was also a weight scale. My son managed to find the button and we determined that I had lost nearly 20 pounds.

Considering that I had been a daily jogger prior to starting this ordeal, and that my starting weight was about 150 pounds, I was not a good candidate for a 15% drop in body weight.

I had not eaten anything for several days, and my last drink of Gatorade - which I had only managed to retain for a few minutes - had been about four days prior.

But the good news was that my body had begun its healing process. I enthusiastically shared news about flatulence and a recent bowel movement with the duty- and staff nurses.

I assumed that they would record this conversation, perhaps make a note in my patient file for the doctor to review... but instead they just smiled and one of them said, "That's good news".

By now, I was starving!

My wife asked whether they could *drip-feed* me, and a lady - I am not sure of her role - said that she would ask the doctor.

But we did not hear from her again.

I figured out a way to get ice delivered to my room.

There was a small rectangular plastic bowl in the room. I asked if they could bring me some ice. Of course, they inquired as to why I would need ice.

I said that I would like to place a few face cloths in the plastic container, cover them with ice, and then use the cold cloths to wipe my face. I would also roll a face cloth and then place the cold cloth on my forehead.

I was not running a temperature, but the room was warm.

Moreover, when they brought me a jug of ice, I placed some of the ice on the face cloth as described above.

And then, I would suck a small ice cube every few minutes.

I filled a plastic cup with ice and cold tap water. Now, I was able to take small sips of ice cold water from time to time, unbeknownst to the nursing police.

Because the amounts of water were so small, any water discharged via the NG tube would not be noticeable. I figured that if they were planning to starve me to death, I would at least prolong my survival for a few days, if I were able to consume some cold water.

My breathing had become labored. Every few minutes I experienced an involuntary gasp for air. My mouth would open, and I would literally gasp, while making an awful rasping sound, for air.

I experienced involuntary abdominal spasms every few minutes. The muscle contractions were symptomatic of starvation, rather than my small bowel obstruction.

Although I am not a medically qualified person, I know the above to be true because the gastric surgeon had previously explained that regular passing of wind and bowel movements meant that my body was healing.

I was healing, but starving!

The hospital's standard care protocols were now slowly killing me.

*****

Day Ten

Monday, April 4th, 2022.

I spent the day lying in bed. When I had no visitors, I read more about Dr. Fauci.

I also started reading *Double Cross*, a New York Times bestseller about the Giancana mob family and their ties to other mobsters, like the Kennedy family.

For most of the day, my wife and both my sons visited, for several hours.

I had surgery scheduled for the next day, early in the morning.

The hospital's resident gastrologist would perform a laparoscopy. This is a surgical procedure in which a fiber-optic instrument is inserted through the abdominal wall to view the organs in the abdomen, or to permit a surgical procedure.

I had no way of knowing whether the nursing staff had informed the good doctor about my healing or recovery in progress, which I had shared with them the previous day.

I had not seen the gastrologist for a few days. The only people who came and went were nurses, doing their standard protocol work – checking vital signs, taking a blood sample, changing a drip, and so on.

Over a period of several days in hospital, not one single hospital employee inquired about my health, requested an update, etc.

For example, a nurse would arrive and say, "I need to check your vitals". She would then proceed to attach her monitoring devices and check my oxygen, blood pressure, pulse, etc., and leave.

An hour later another nurse would arrive, check the drip, replace it if needed, and leave.

The examples above represent standard care protocols.

This is not patient care… but rather just *room service* in exchange for billing the patient for *healthcare services*.

I asked for water.

As mentioned, I was literally starving.

They said: "No, you are NPO."

NPO means "nothing by mouth," derived from the Latin *nil per os*.

I was convinced that they were killing me slowly.

Day Eleven

Tuesday, April 5th, 2022.

Early in the morning I was taken to pre-op. There, the medical orderlies prepared me for surgery.

They are experts who knew what they were doing. However, at this stage of my in-patient tenure, I was confident that I no longer needed surgery.

The procedure the surgeon eventually performed was a *diagnostic laparoscopy*. A diagnostic laparoscopy is a procedure that, for example, allows a doctor to look directly at the contents of the abdomen or pelvis.

He also billed for a procedure coded as "Release Small Intestine, Percutaneous Endoscopic Approach".

Translated into simple terms, for my procedure:

Release (by force vs. surgically) in this example means pushing and prodding the small intestine to dislodge a blockage.

Percutaneous describes small incisions (vs. open surgery) that are made, done, or effected through the skin.

And an endoscopic procedure involves inserting a long, flexible tube (called an endoscope) with a tiny camera on the end. The endoscope allows a doctor to examine the stomach and the beginning of the small intestine (duodenum).

*****

A few hours after my pre-op and subsequent surgical adventure, I *woke up* in a post-op care room, and was taken back to my hospital room.

Upon arrival, I experienced an overwhelming sense of happiness and relief.

I had survived the entire ordeal!

More importantly, I saw my wife's beautiful, smiling face. Smiling despite her obvious concern for my wellbeing over the previous ten days, and the related stress she had to endure.

To help make things even better, both my sons and one daughter-in-law were there, at my bedside, waiting to welcome me back from surgery.

*****

The previous night, prior to going into surgery that Tuesday morning, I had hardly slept due to trepidation caused by the pending and upcoming surgical procedure.

Now, post-surgery, my family left a little while later and I was able to get some sleep.

By that evening I was well rested.

I visually checked the plastic container that was attached to the other end of the NG tube.

It was empty.

That was a good sign.

It meant that there were no gastric juices or liquids to drain from my empty stomach. In turn, this meant that my body was basically functioning as intended.

Gastric juices were moving from my stomach into the small intestine instead of being extracted via the suction tube.

During the night hours I was more awake than asleep. I kept checking the plastic container attached to the other end of my NG tube.

It was still empty.

I decided to discharge myself the next day.

Doing so would be *against medical advice* (AMA).

At 4 AM I got up and washed.

Then I removed the NG tube.

I had previously served in the South African Army as an operational (or Ops) medic. As a result, extracting the tube was a simple procedure, uncomfortable, but not scary at all.

With the tube removed I was able to wash and shave my face for the first time in more than a week.

Getting cleaned up helps one to become instantly more upbeat as you can likely observe from the picture below.

Conversely, a twenty-pound weight loss, unkempt hair, further complemented by scraggly, ten-day-old facial stubble… collectively create a distinctive *homeless* and somewhat desperate look.

Within a few minutes, I had been able to transform myself visually from starving hospital patient - with an NG tube protruding from my right nostril - to a cleaner version of myself, and somewhat presentable despite being emaciated.

Of course, I also removed my drip, along with its various attachments.

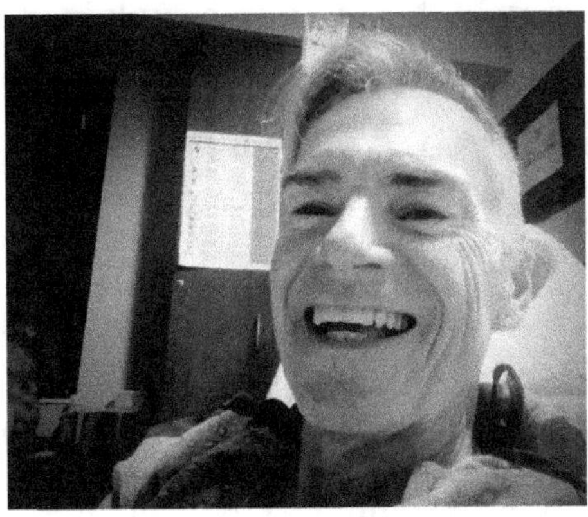

What I was unable to do, was add back the 20 pounds of weight loss from nearly two weeks of starvation.

This was obviously not entirely the fault of the hospital's staff, but they had played a leading role.

*****

By the time the duty nurse came into my room the next morning at around 6 AM, she gasped at my appearance. I was sitting on a lounge chair, fully dressed, cleaned up, tubes removed, and ready to depart.

Her first words were, "You removed the tube!"

She asked me what I was doing. I said that I would be leaving after breakfast, as soon as they had brought me some food and drink.

"You're NPO", she said.

I countered by saying that I was literally starving. I added that if they did not bring me food, I would simply have to go to the hospital's cafeteria to buy something to eat.

Somewhat exasperated, the day nurse explained that she was not allowed to give me any food.

Within a few minutes I had a group of about six or seven nurses and staff milling in and around my room and my doorway.

The duty nurse verbally scolded, warned and threatened me (about leaving AMA), instructed me to wait for the doctor to arrive around lunchtime, warned me that the medical insurance company would not pay any of my bills, and more.

Her dire warning that "the medical insurance company would not help to pay my bills" is somewhat related to the events described above about in- and/or out-of-network providers... but more about that later.

I found it somewhat interesting that not a single staff member expressed any care or concern about my health or welfare.

No-one asked me how I was feeling at that time. Nor did they inquire about who might assist me if I discharged myself and needed help.

Their only concern seemed to be my imminent departure without their permission.

An in-patient client - or maybe I should just call myself a human *Automatic Banking Machine* - was threatening to leave and walk out the door.

Any such proposed exit would arrest a lucrative, recurring source of revenue for the hospital!

Side Note:

Billing statements I started receiving post-departure soon helped me to better understand why hospitals might be reluctant to discharge patients.

*****

In the context of the recent *Covid-19 pandemic*, my personal experience helped me to better understand why so many people went to hospital in the United States for Covid, and then died soon thereafter.

The U.S. Food and Drug Administration-approved treatment regimen of Remdesivir and ventilation appeared to have done more damage than good.

Remdesivir is sold under the brand name Veklury. It was developed, and is marketed, as a broad-spectrum antiviral medication by biopharmaceutical company Gilead Sciences.

On August 14, 2021, Oxford Academic published a study titled *"Remdesivir and Mortality in Patients With Coronavirus Disease 2019"* opening with this paragraph:

"The impact of remdesivir (RDV) on mortality rates in

> *coronavirus disease 2019 (COVID-19) is controversial, and the mortality effect in subgroups of baseline disease severity has been incompletely explored."*

I will refrain from discussing this controversial topic, save to say that more people per capita died in the United States *with Covid*, than in any other country. A primary reason for this unfortunate turn of events was the inclusion of deaths flagged *with Covid* in U.S. all-cause mortality stats.

Other reasons include absolute, epic failure of government agencies regarding any/all alternative treatments, their stifling and ongoing censorship of all expert counter-opinion, collusion between corrupt *big-pharma* and bureaucrats on the take, ineffective vaccines, and more.

Day Twelve

On the morning of April 6th, 2022, I arrived home at around 11 AM.

During my hospital stay, I had promised myself that if I were to survive and walk out of hospital one day, I would treat myself to a root beer float.

I realize that this might sound ridiculous, but perhaps not unlike a pregnant woman experiencing some crazy cravings, I could hardly wait to have the drink above.

The sips of root beer and nibbles of vanilla ice cream from the float were simply delicious!

During my absence from home, my family had purchased some high energy protein drink powders that could be blended with milk (for extra protein), and a small blender.

My diet would be mostly liquids for the next few days. I consumed large amounts of soup (with small bits of bread added), puddings, ice cream, and various energy drinks.

About two days later I had recovered sufficiently to start eating solid food. Initially, my solid food diet was limited to adding a slice of bread and bits of chicken to a bowl of soup.

Soon thereafter, I started eating starches like potatoes and rice, and easily digestible protein, like ground beef.

Within days I started getting stronger and I had regained a few lost pounds.

*****

PART FOUR

The Negotiations

CHAPTER 8: THE GREAT AMERICAN HEALTHCARE BILLING SCAM

In case you missed the previous chapters, here is a one-paragraph summary:

Once upon a time, during a period spanning about two weeks, I went to a local emergency room three times, and spent a total of four nights in a hospital room. I received a variety of first-world healthcare treatments and services, delivered by experts in a variety of different healthcare disciplines.

The various service providers above submitted all their invoices to my medical insurance company for processing and payment.

The grand total: About $180,000 (*updated 2024*)

A four-day in-patient hospital stay: $100,000.

The balance: ER visits and subcontractor services.

One, single visit and treatment at the local emergency room, described in the previous chapter in *Day One*, was billed at over $10,000. This did not include the examining doctor's fees which were billed separately.

Various additional charges from subcontractors and service agencies (lab work, x-rays, etc.) are included in the *big number* above. They all submitted invoices individually and separately to my medical insurance company.

All the service providers above and the local regional medical health center (located nearest to my home), were out-of-network according to my insurer. This simply meant that I - in my personal capacity - would be liable for the entire amount billed.

You might recall that my mentioning above that I had not selected the hospital. I ended up there because on *Day One*, an ambulance had picked me up at home after I had called 911.

The medics delivered me to the nearest ER, as one would expect. Anyway, as a patient in the back of an ambulance, doubled-over in excruciating abdominal pain, our proposed destination was the least of my worries!

At that time, I did not think to ask the medics where they were taking me. Arguably, I was not thinking at all at that time!

When I returned to the same ER a few days later, I also did not check whether the hospital was in-network. I had no way of knowing that the ER doctor would be admitting me to the adjoining hospital.

To be fair, even if I had known, I would probably not have checked the hospital's in- or out-of-network status, simply because I had never imagined that the hospital nearest to my home would be out-of-network.

For the benefit of people located outside of the USA, healthcare providers designated as out-of-network providers implies that the patient will be personally responsible for the entire bill.

In my case, just as a reminder... $180,000.

*****

Under Obamacare, no medical insurance company may refuse to provide an Explanation of Benefits (EOB), nor refuse processing and payment for Emergency Room services.

However, they are within their rights to dispute the patient's choice to go to an emergency room rather than, for example, a walk-in clinic.

So, we can start the billing journey with this example:

Date(s) of Service	Benefit Description	Proc Code	Amount Billed	Excluded Amount	Bright Discount	Co-Pay Amount	Deductible Amount	Amount Allowed	Paid At	What we will pay
03/26-03/26/22	HOS MISC FEE	00000	392.00	0.00	311.11	0.00	80.89	80.89	100%	0.00
03/26-03/26/22	LABORATORY	36415	3,568.00	0.00	2,831.70	0.00	736.30	736.30	100%	0.00
03/26-03/26/22	EMER RM ILL	96361	5,419.00	0.00	4,300.71	0.00	785.52	1,118.29	100%	332.77
03/26-03/26/22	DIAGNOSTIC	93005	751.00	0.00	596.02	0.00	0.00	154.98	100%	154.98
03/26-03/26/22	INTEREST	00000	1.28	0.00	0.00	0.00	0.00	1.28	0%	1.28
	Column Totals		10,131.28	0.00	8,039.54	0.00	1,602.71	2,091.74		489.03

From the snapshot above, we can observe a few interesting factoids.

The hospital's original invoice amount was $10,131.

The medical insurance company discount, despite disputing overall liability, was $8,039.

The deductible amount that I would have to pay was $1,602.

The medical insurance company paid $489.

As mentioned above, an insurer cannot legally refuse to pay for an ER visit unless they could prove, for example, that the ER visit had been unnecessary. In this case, the insurer's offer to pay their share of $489 was probably significantly less costly than paying to legally defend a refusal to pay for services, should that have been necessary.

And finally, the medical center accepted a percentage equal to about 20% of their total ER invoice amount, in full and final settlement.

This is how medical and healthcare providers invoice their services in the United States. They know and understand that they will not be paid whatever the charged amount is, but they persist with the billing scam anyway.

This would be no different to your local pizza takeout billing you $150 for a family-sized pizza, and then accepting an offer of $30 in full and final settlement.

How can I be sure that the hospital will accept an eighty percent reduction of their invoice as a full settlement?

Because that is exactly what happened!

The hospital received $489 from the insurance company, and invoiced me for the remaining balance ($1,602.71) that was due:

Account Activity

Total Charges:	$10,130.00
Ins. Payments & Adjustments:	$487.75
Insurance Pending:	$0.00
Patient Payments:	$0.00
Current Account Balance:	$1,602.71
Monthly Payment Amount:	$0.00
I Owe:	$1,602.71

All the examples immediately above relate to my first visit to ER, on Day One.

You might be thinking, "That is not too bad. Settling a $10,000 bill for $1,600 out of pocket."

However, the invoice above is only the hospital's direct charge for one ER visit. The expert doctor who misdiagnosed my condition originally, would also submit his invoice.

Date(s) of Service	Benefit Description	Proc Code	Amount Billed	Excluded Amount	Bright Discount	Co-Pay Amount	Deductible Amount	Amount Allowed	Paid At	What we will pay
03/26-03/26/22	EMERG VISIT	99285	2,054.00	0.00	1,815.96	0.00	238.04	238.04	100%	0.00
03/26-03/26/22	PROF COMP	93010	96.00	0.00	85.13	0.00	10.87	10.87	100%	0.00
	Column Totals		2,150.00	0.00	1,901.09	0.00	248.91	248.91		0.00

I owe: 248.91

What we will pay   0.00

Reimbursement is based on the regulations under the No Surprises Act or applicable state law. Member is not responsible and cannot be balanced billed for covered out of network services beyond allowed amount. For more

The ER Doctor sent a separate bill for his consultation.

In this example the insurer reduced the $2,150 invoiced amount by $1901 and pegged my personal liability at $248 due for payment to the provider.

But there is a note added to the EOB snapshot above:

> *Reimbursement is based on the regulations under the No Surprises Act or applicable state law. Member is not responsible and cannot be balanced billed for covered out of network services beyond allowed amount.*

This additional comment is another favorable condition added via Obamacare for the protection of patients who are invoiced huge, unexpected amounts for services delivered, that they were unaware of purchasing.

In the example immediately above, I paid the doctor - via his outsourced billing service - the $248 due by me.

"How did the doctor's billing service respond to the transaction, you might wonder?"

I will help you out.

They simply resubmitted the invoice for payment again. As if nothing had happened to change their minds. Or, as if they had not received any payment at all.

In other words, the patient billing saga ends when the provider decides that they have exhausted all options that can be employed to extract money from *victims*.

*****

Here is an example of a *big hospital bill* for $66,202:

Date(s) of Service	Benefit Description	Proc Code	Amount Billed	Excluded Amount	Bright Discount	Co-Pay Amount	Deductible Amount	Amount Allowed	Paid At	What we will pay
04/03-04/06/22	ROOM & BOARD	00000	9,594.00	9,594.00	0.00	0.00	0.00	0.00	0%	0.00
04/03-04/06/22	I/P ANC FEES	00000	36,321.00	36,321.00	0.00	0.00	0.00	0.00	0%	0.00
04/03-04/06/22	I/P ANC FEES	00000	5,131.00	5,131.00	0.00	0.00	0.00	0.00	0%	0.00
04/03-04/06/22	I/P ANC FEES	00000	12,793.00	12,793.00	0.00	0.00	0.00	0.00	0%	0.00
04/03-04/06/22	I/P ANC FEES	00000	2,363.00	2,363.00	0.00	0.00	0.00	0.00	0%	0.00
	Column Totals		66,202.00	66,202.00	0.00	0.00	0.00	0.00		0.00

A hospital bill for a 3-day in-patient room & care services, April 3-6, 2022

And the insurer's note below the amounts invoiced:

(Line 1-$9,594.00)(Line 2-$36,321.00)(Line 3-$5,131.00)(Line 4-$12,793.00)(Line 5-$2,363.00)SERVICES RENDERED BY A NON-PARTICIPATING PROVIDER ARE NOT COVERED. IF PROVIDER IS IN NETWORK UNDER A DIFFERENT TAX IDENTIFICATION/NPI NUMBER, THE CLAIM MUST BE RESUBMITTED WITH THAT TAX IDENTIFICATION/NPI NUMBER FOR CONSIDERATION.**** PLEASE REFER TO THE LIMITATIONS/ EXCLUSIONS SECTION OF THE CERTIFICATE OF COVERAGE.
Services rendered by an out-of-network provider are not covered.

A note added by the insurance company, rejecting the entire claim

Because the hospital is out-of-network and the invoice does not relate to emergency room services, the entire invoiced amount is my responsibility as per their added note, above.

If this were your debt to pay, you might be asking yourself, "What would I do?"

I will do my best to answer this question in the next chapters. If you add my other large invoice for $34,000 (*image below*) to the invoice above, you arrive at the total billing of more than $100,000 due for a hospital stay, along with the related services that I mentioned earlier.

Date(s) of Service	Benefit Description	Proc Code	Amount Billed	Excluded Amount	Bright Discount	Co-Pay Amount	Deductible Amount	Amount Allowed	Paid At	What we will pay
04/01-04/02/22	ROOM & BOARD	00000	3,198.00	3,198.00	0.00	0.00	0.00	0.00	0%	0.00
04/01-04/02/22	I/P ANC FEES	00000	6,027.00	6,027.00	0.00	0.00	0.00	0.00	0%	0.00
04/01-04/02/22	I/P ANC FEES	00000	4,803.00	4,803.00	0.00	0.00	0.00	0.00	0%	0.00
04/01-04/02/22	I/P ANC FEES	00000	7,372.00	7,372.00	0.00	0.00	0.00	0.00	0%	0.00
04/01-04/02/22	I/P ANC FEES	00000	12,793.00	12,793.00	0.00	0.00	0.00	0.00	0%	0.00
04/01-04/02/22	I/P ANC FEES	00000	437.00	437.00	0.00	0.00	0.00	0.00	0%	0.00
	Column Totals		34,630.00	34,630.00	0.00	0.00	0.00	0.00		0.00

A hospital bill for 1-day in-patient room & care services, April 1-2, 2022

*****

CHAPTER 9:
BALLOONING
HEALTHCARE COSTS

On average, annual healthcare expenditures are about $10,000 per person in the United States.

This is more than twice the rate of other industrialized nations. Some insurance service providers estimate U.S. healthcare costs of more than $3.3 trillion per year.

A large amount of the total healthcare billings is settled by medical insurance companies, after they are reduced by some steep pre-negotiated discounts for in-network service providers.

But estimates are that more than $350 billion dollars are spent directly by the end user or patient in terms of out-of-pocket medical expenses.

More than 1% of the U.S. population (more than 3 million people) are hit hardest. They end up spending over $20,000 out-of-pocket annually on healthcare.

According to some analysts, nearly 20 million Americans are forced into bankruptcy (or outright poverty) because of unaffordable health care expenses.

Anyone who might have a medical bill that they are unable to pay must know that - even though it might feel like it - they are not alone.

Peter Kaison's Health Systems Tracker provides a treasure trove of information, like this graph below:

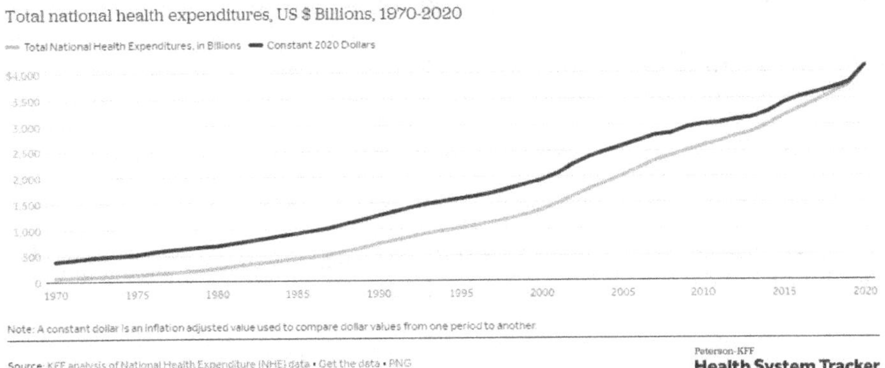

Patients get squeezed for three primary reasons. These include hospital price gouging (most common), incorrectly denied insurance claims, and hospital billing "errors".

Students and analysts of the U.S. healthcare billing system - using Center for Medicare and Medicaid Services (CMS) estimates - show that hospitals frequently charge more than four times their own costs for care services.

But insurance companies and hospitals negotiate discounts off the set prices upfront. That is the primary delta between the in- and out-of-network prices billed.

Initially, consumers are charged more than 3 times what a typical U.S. insurance company will eventually pay a hospital.

Even if you think you have a great health insurance plan, you might go to a hospital and expect any treatments you receive to be covered.

But much like me, you could receive an enormous medical bill from the hospital a few months later. The hospital might claim - correctly too - that your insurance company denied coverage for services that were provided out-of-network, even by subcontractors that you were blissfully unaware of.

Nearly 20% of in-network insurance claims end up being denied in the U.S., and almost none of them are appealed.

Hospitals tend to be good about appealing insurance denied claims (63% success rate), while insurance companies are far more likely to say no to consumers (14% success rate).

Healthcare insurance companies use confusing jargon, codes and set up roadblocks to make clients simply *give up*. And unfortunately, the average consumer just gives up.

*****

Nearly thirteen percent of all medical bills are erroneous in some way or another, according to a NerdWallet study on the medical debt crisis.

Some billing analysts estimate that as much as seventy percent of hospital bills contain errors. Of course, these errors are almost always in favor of hospitals rather than patients.

Frequent errors are an outcome of highly complex billing systems. Hospitals often charge patients for the same thing multiple times, charge for services they had not provided, or engage in *balance billing* practices because hospitals - despite their own erroneous and exuberant billing practices - frequently accuse insurance companies of not *paying their fair share*.

To date, about half of U.S. states have passed laws protecting consumers from balance billing and there are bipartisan efforts in Congress to curb this practice. But hospitals have not stopped their balance billing practices.

*****

An overwhelming stack of medical bills, Explanation of Benefits (EOB) provided by insurance companies to clients, and related documents, are burdensome and confusing.

For the average patient, it also appears as if hospitals and insurance companies are intentionally making things as difficult as possible for the clients to understand.

As I had illustrated in my examples above, it is common for patients to receive multiple bills. These may be sent to you from the ambulance service, a consulting doctor you might not recall speaking with, the hospital's emergency room, a lab that had to analyze your blood or urine tests, etc.

These are all separate companies (subcontractors) who bill patients separately for the services they provide.

This is also true from the perspective of a hospital when billing patients who had never been to that hospital.

Using my hospital visit as an example; the Billing FAQ section on their website offers this statement:

"... the Medical Center provides a wide range of medically related services for independent clinics, area physicians and other hospitals. For example, a pediatrician or health center may refer lab work to ... Medical Center for testing or analysis. When this occurs, the bill for the lab services will come from ... Medical Center."
(Name of facility intentionally omitted above)

For patients - or shall we say victims - it is important not to become overwhelmed. Take a deep breath and then take a medical bill, one at a time, and start breaking it down to ensure that you understand each part.

The first concept to understand is that your bill includes a *rack rate* or *chargemaster rate* for the healthcare services provided.

Perhaps more familiar terms might be that the bill illustrates the provider's *gross charges* or *full rack rate* ...before any discounts.

These are also the rates that hospitals charge to uninsured patients. The prices listed on hospital bills have little bearing on reality and are not the prices insurance companies end up paying.

Very often, the charges are completely made up, but more importantly, you should never pay the prices as per the bill.

Some people in the medical industry literally call the prices on hospital bills *the sucker price*. Most hospitals know that no one ever pays this rate, and neither should you!

Insurance discounts (or adjustments) on medical bills represent a pre-negotiated discount between an insurer and a hospital. You will only see or receive such an adjustment on your bill if you have insurance.

Always request a detailed, itemized bill from the hospital.

Once you have that itemized bill you will be able to compare it to the insurance company's "Explanation of Benefits" (EOBs).

*****

The Balance or *Patient Portion* is everything that's left over after all adjustments and insurance company payments have been deducted from the total amount of the bill.

This represents the bottom-line of what you owe the hospital. If you have medical insurance, the Patient Portion is often called the copay or deductible.

The Balance is the gross total of billed charges less any insurance adjustments less any insurance payments.

Here is an example from my personal file:

Amount Billed	Excluded Amount	Bright Discount	Co-Pay Amount	Deductible Amount	Amount Allowed	At
2,054.00	0.00	1,815.96	0.00	238.04	238.04	100%
96.00	0.00	85.13	0.00	10.87	10.87	100%
2,150.00	0.00	1,901.09	0.00	248.91	248.91	

Balance Billing Example: Patient Portion

In the snapshot above, the provider billed $2,150 for services. The insurance company discount was $1,901.09, leaving a Balance Billed to the patient of $248.91.

The example above illustrates a provider billing an amount that is nearly ten times greater than the pre-negotiated insurance rate.

Amount Billed	Excluded Amount	Bright Discount	Co-Pay Amount	Deductible Amount	Amount Allowed	At	What we will pay
392.00	0.00	311.11	0.00	80.89	80.89	100%	0.00
3,568.00	0.00	2,831.70	0.00	736.30	736.30	100%	0.00
5,419.00	0.00	4,300.71	0.00	785.52	1,118.29	100%	332.77
751.00	0.00	596.02	0.00	0.00	154.98	100%	154.98
1.28	0.00	0.00	0.00	0.00	1.28	0%	1.28
10,131.28	0.00	8,039.54	0.00	1,602.71	2,091.74		489.03

Balance Billing Example: Patient & Insurer Portion

In the snapshot immediately above, I added the "What we will pay" column on the right, showing the insurer's payment contribution.

The Amount Billed is $10,131.28. The insurance discount is $8,039.54. The Deductible (Patient Portion) is $1,602.71. The insurance company paid $489.03.

The example above illustrates a provider billing an amount nearly five times greater than the final payment they expect to receive from the insurance company and the patient together; or using rounded numbers, $2,000 to settle a $10,000 bill.

It seems as if a few hospitals have realized that patients are more likely to pay bills if they understand what they're being charged for. Companies like Simplee are building software to help hospitals streamline their billing processes.

For all the parties in the healthcare billing scam, making things as clear as possible would be an important step to ensuring that patients stop getting ripped off, and that reasonable charges are paid.

The insurance company will provide clients with an Explanation of Benefits (EOB) document. The EOB will help to bring clarity to costs and coverages.

It is critical for people with hospital bills to compare the hospital's itemized bill with the insurer's EOB.

There are line items that patients should become familiar with.

These include the service/product that shows the type of medical service delivered. It might be a description and/or include a CPT or HCPCS code.

The charges that will be your responsibility is often presented in one or a combination of three descriptions:

Copay is a shared payment for services provided. Sometimes the copay is a fixed and relatively small amount (e.g., $20 copay for a doctor's visit). Sometimes the copay is a percentage of the total bill (e.g., 20%).

Many insurance plans require that clients cover a certain amount of expenses before benefits kick in. This is called a *deductible*.

In my personal examples shared as a patient, my deductible was

$8,700. That meant that I was personally responsible for the first $8,700 of any/all medical bills before my insurance company would pay anything.

However, discounts on services that the insurance company negotiated with the hospital should still apply if the hospital was in-network. If the hospital was out-of-network (as in my example), I would be responsible for 100% of the bill.

It is critically important for insured patients to determine whether their medical service providers are in- or out-of-network, BEFORE agreeing to any services.

Otherwise, like me, you might be responsible for the entire bill, and would have to negotiate with the providers, or hire someone to do this on your behalf, for a hefty fee.

Of course, people being taken to ER in the back of an ambulance very seldom get to choose the destination. That is why - under the Obamacare legislation passed - ER visits cannot be dismissed or categorized as out-of-network by insurers.

Below you will find a short glossary of common verbiage on EOB documents received from your insurance company:

Coinsurance is a percentage of the bill that you pay after you've met the deductible. The rest would be paid by your insurance company. If, for example, your medical insurance plan has a 20% coinsurance requirement you will have responsibility for that percentage of the bill. Your insurance company will cover the remaining 80%.

The *Provider* is the healthcare service provider (e.g., a hospital).

Their *Amount Billed* is the initial amount they charged for your visit (aka a *Chargemaster Rate*). It must correspond with the charges on your itemized hospital bill and will typically be significantly higher than the *Allowed Amount* (below).

The discount off the Chargemaster Rate that your insurance

company has negotiated with a hospital is referred to as the *Plan Discount*. This is also often called an "insurance adjustment" or "contractual amount".

The amount that the healthcare provider is allowed to charge for their services (versus the Amount Billed), is called the *Allowed Amount* or *Allowed Charges*. These charges are based on the insurance company's contract with the provider.

Insurance Coverage or *Paid by Insurer* is the amount of money that the insurance company paid the hospital and should be the same amount as the Insurance Payment on the hospital bill. Adding this amount to Your Responsibility (how much you owe) should equal Allowed Charges.

*****

A few interesting data points, in summary:

Annual expenditure on healthcare in the U.S. is spiraling out of control. Millions of Americans are paying way more than they should for out-of-pocket costs, for medical bills.

Most of the time, the contributors to excessive out-of-pocket medical costs are (a) incorrectly denied insurance claims, (b) hospital price gouging, and (c) hospital billing "errors".

Insurer EOB documents, itemized medical bills, and other medically-related documents are designed to be confusing. It appears as if hospitals and insurance companies are intentionally making things as difficult to decipher as possible.

When you receive a hospital bill, you should never pay the full Billed Charges, or Chargemaster Rate.

Insurance companies all negotiate a discount (the contractual discount) with hospitals to come up with a new price (the allowed amount).

If you have insurance, make sure you are only paying the allowed amount. If you do not have insurance, be sure to read the next chapter so that you can learn how to figure out a good price to pay.

*****

CHAPTER 10: HOW MUCH SHOULD I PAY?

There are a few things you need to know, and a few simple steps to consider when negotiating a hospital bill. In this chapter, we will provide some guidance and tips.

*****

For starters, gather the right information and make sure that you understand all the relevant documents related to your bills.

Hospitals do not typically provide itemized bills, but they are required by law to do so if you ask them directly.

Call the hospital's customer service number. Expect to hold on for about an hour while listening to piped music and occasional reminders that *your call is important* and to *hold on for the next available customer service representative.*

Author's tip:

The biller's customer service line might have an option like, "to pay your bill, press 3". Always select this option because you will be connected quickly.

The person on the other side of the line is also a customer service representative. The provider is simply prioritizing and/or connecting people who are offering to pay their bills… first.

When you eventually connect, ask the representative for an itemized bill. Say, "I would like an itemized bill."

Itemized bills list line-by-line charges and their associated revenue codes (internal codes hospitals use to determine their charge), CPT or HCPCS code (used to identify what services were provided), and charges for each line item.

Your insurance company will send you an Explanation of Benefits (EOB), or make it available online, or both. You can also call your insurance company and ask them to send it to you. If you do not have insurance, ignore this document.

*****

Review and compare your billing detail and EOB for billing issues or errors.

Note that hospitals charge consumers, on average, about four times their actual costs and about three times the price that insurance companies pay for the same service.

If you do not have insurance your bill is almost certainly inflated. Every time. The hospital will nearly always charge you their rack rates. This means that you are almost certainly a victim of price-gouging.

If you have insurance but the EOB has no reference to a *Plan Discount*, or if the Plan Discount is for a very small amount relative to the total charges, you are most certainly being price-gouged.

Call the insurance company. Ask them to walk you through the bill. Confirm that the Plan Discount amount is correct.

People are often too embarrassed, shy, or afraid to negotiate hospital bills, but this is exactly what you should do.

Hospitals are quite used to clients calling them to negotiate their bills, or even to offer them a payment offer in full and final settlement of an outstanding bill.

Anyway, hospitals prefer this direct approach by clients. It is more desirable for them than having to send overdue bills to collection agencies.

Ask the hospital to reduce the price they are charging you, to a more reasonable amount.

If you have done your homework, you can even suggest an amount that is in line with the amounts insurance companies pay, rather than the ridiculously inflated *Chargemaster Rate*.

Do not call the general customer service line to demand a discount. Service representatives will usually suggest that you apply for financial aid or set up a payment plan. They are not authorized to lower your bill.

You need to do a little more homework first!

To start, you need to build your case. Once you have all the information ready (your business case), you can submit a settlement request. Be prepared to start negotiating if your settlement offer is not accepted.

Asking for a discount is often not enough. You need to provide the hospital with a strong reason to accept a lower amount.

You need to demonstrate or convince them that the amount they billed will create a financial hardship for you and your family.

Arguing financial hardship gets easier and more believable as bills get larger. There is no need for you to provide detailed financial records. Rather share that you have received multiple bills related to your hospital stay and/or procedure, if this is true, and that everything together makes it very difficult or impossible for you to be able to pay.

You should confidently demonstrate that prices charged are far out of the ordinary. With a little homework under your belt, you will be able to compare what ordinary and/or reasonable prices might be, based on insurance rates, for example.

If you want to demonstrate that a particular line item or charge is out of the ordinary, you will need to do a bit of research.

Look up Medicare reimbursable pricing or sign up for a free trial of Find-A-Code online. With the latter you can enter an HCPCS/CPT code from your itemized bill and compare the Medicare reimbursable rate.

In the U.S., insurance companies generally pay 1.5-3x the Medicare reimbursable, so you can use that range for your initial offer.

A Google search of the "charge/cost ratio [hospital name]" is a bit of a long shot, but you could try that route to find something informative related to your hospital.

Once you have built a solid case, you can consider submitting a settlement request. This would be a starting point for any negotiation. It is also a good way for you to steer the conversation with the hospital representative away from suggesting a payment plan.

You need to write a settlement request letter. The letter will give the hospital something to respond to. More importantly, it will force them to start talking about the price rather than about payment plans and/or suggesting that you should apply for financial aid.

When you write a settlement offer letter, be sure to include the following details and information:

Your account number(s).
Your name and address.
The amount outstanding on your bill.
The amount you are offering to pay for their services.
Some high-level details about your offer (e.g., based on
Medicare Reimbursable rates or Charge/Cost Ratios).
State that you will pay immediately if they accept your offer
(if possible). This will encourage them to accept the offer.
And a short paragraph to thank the hospital for their services.

Proofread your letter - or ask someone else to review it for you - to ensure the information is correct and that there are no spelling or grammar errors.

Make your offer look professional!

*****

Here is a copy of the offer letter I had sent to my hospital:

Thank you for reviewing and considering my request for assistance!

The bills received for the ABC Medical Center's Services - in addition to numerous other bills received for services delivered during my visits to ER and as an in-patient - collectively place my family in a position of considerable financial hardship.

I am willing to make a settlement offer of up to 20% of the balances due to the ABC Medical Center. This would amount to approximately $20,000. Please advise me if this is acceptable. If your organization accepts my offer in full-and-final settlement of all bills due, I will do my best to make that payment within 5 business days from receipt of your acceptance letter.

What happened?

I did not request to be taken to ABC's ER facility. An ambulance took me there on March 26, 2022. At the time of my initial visit, the ER doctor misdiagnosed my condition as food poisoning, and I returned home.

My condition deteriorated over the next few days. I was in a very weak physical state due to extreme abdominal pain, a lack of nutrition, and ongoing vomiting when I returned to the same ER department on March 31, 2022.

This time the consulting doctor diagnosed my condition as a "High Grade Small Bowel Obstruction" and admitted me to the hospital as an in-patient.

As requested, I informed the various staff members that my insurer is XYZ. No-one advised me that the hospital located nearest to my home - and the ER where I had originally been taken to by ambulance - was "out of network".

At the time, I had no way of knowing; no staff members from ABC suggested that I should inquire; and I also had no idea that many of the Medical Center's services would have been out-of-network anyway, even if the hospital itself were in-network.

This is a summary of events, explaining how I ended up being "uninsured" and the recipient of medical bills totaling more than $150,000.

I sincerely appreciate the care and attention I received while I was an in-patient at your hospital! Your staff members were kind, efficient, and their expertise inspired confidence.

Please let me know your response to my offer above at your earliest convenience.

*****

When you are ready, call the client services number on your hospital bill and ask how you can submit a settlement request. They will provide a fax number, email address, or post office mailing address.

Many hospitals will accept settlement requests, but billing department representatives are trained and required to redirect you to their other, preferred payment methods. Be firm asking how you can submit a settlement request until they tell you how to go about doing this.

Depending on how you submitted the letter (i.e., email or surface mail), call the hospital within the next day or few days to confirm receipt of your letter and ask how long it will take for them to respond.

You may have to call back multiple times to confirm receipt of your settlement offer... but just keep going!

Customer service representatives might say that they did not receive it, that they lost it, etc. Do not be deterred. Be patient and persistent.

Check the status of your settlement request until you receive a response. As a rule, hospitals will only respond if you keep *pushing* the billing department for a response.

If the hospital accepts your settlement offer, congratulations!

Now all you will need to do is pay the bill.

What if they decline your settlement offer?

This would be the start of some required negotiation. Ask them for the reason why they declined your offer. Whatever their response, ask them to provide it in writing along with their settlement counteroffer.

You may need to ask to speak to a supervisor to make your case over the phone. It might end up being a long process of asking for a discount, being declined, and then trying again.

*****

Insurance companies might refuse to pay for a medical procedure even though you went to an in-network hospital.

This is often due to one of two reasons: the medical procedure was not covered under your insurance policy; or the medical services provided were not for a medical emergency.

The Explanation of Benefits (EOB) from your insurance company should clearly state both if your claim was denied AND the reason for your denial. It's important to note the reason for denial, as that determines the best path to appealing your claim.

The EOB might include explanations like these:

Services rendered by an out-of-network provider are not covered.

Reimbursement is based on the regulations under the No Surprises Act or applicable state law.

Member is not responsible and cannot be balanced billed for covered out of network services beyond allowed amount.

If you have medical insurance, and the insurance company rejected your claim, you can submit an appeal. Appealing insurance claim denials requires attention to detail, good record-keeping, and once again being patient, yet persistent.

Many health insurance companies have deadlines for filing appeals (e.g., 180 days from date of claim). Make sure to act fast to get the appeal out the door and into the hands of the insurance company, as soon as possible once you have collected and reviewed all the relevant information.

Claims denied because of clerical errors (e.g., a misspelled name, wrong insurance ID, etc.) are relatively straightforward and easy to fix.

These can usually be settled easily with a phone call to a customer service representative. They may ask you to refile your claim. Make sure that your refiled claim is correct before submitting it, and you should be all set.

*****

If your insurance claim was denied for a different reason - e.g., the treatment received was not a covered procedure, or not a medical emergency - you can consider the following actions below.

Make sure you understand their processes and required paperwork. There is a lot of work involved in filing an appeal, so be sure to track everything carefully.

Look for the paperwork and process for filing an appeal in the insurance company's online portal. If you cannot find it, call the customer service number, and ask.

Write yourself a step-by-step process guideline and make a checklist of the paperwork they require.

You can work with your doctor and the hospital to gather any relevant evidence required. This might include a referral from your doctor to another medical provider, medical history records to show a treatment or procedure was a medical necessity, a note from your doctor affirming medical necessity, etc.

If you believe that your procedure should be a covered procedure, include an explanation of this along with a note from the doctor or hospital.

Once you have gathered all the evidence and completed their required forms, you can submit your appeal.

Read the claim form carefully and follow each step exactly as it is written. Mistakes can cause your appeal to be denied due to clerical error, forcing you to go through the process of filling out everything again.

You might need to call your insurance company every couple of weeks to check on the status of your claim. Appeals can take time, but you can ask them for an expected timeline for processing your appeal.

*****

As described previously, the difference between the amount your insurance company paid and a hospital's Chargemaster Rates, is called *Balance Billing*.

If an insurance company negotiated special rates with a hospital, as part of that agreement, the hospital may not charge those insured the difference between their standard rates and the negotiated rates.

There are two types of balance billing: In-Network and Out-of-Network.

In-Network Balance Billing occurs when the insurance company and the hospital have a contract defining a set rate for services, and the hospital attempts to bill you extra on top of that defined rate, which their contract disallows.

Out-of-Network Balance Billing occurs when you go "out-of-network" for a medical treatment. That is, the medical service provider does not have a negotiated price agreement with your insurance company.

In these cases, the insurance company determines on its own what it will pay the hospital for these services, or if they will pay anything at all.

There is no contract stating that the hospital cannot charge the patient the difference between what the insurance company paid and the hospital charge master rate.

Patients can identify this situation by comparing the Explanation of Benefits (EOB) from the insurance company with the itemized bill, sent to the patient by the hospital. The EOB will inform the patient that the healthcare provider is in- or out-of-network.

Also, if the numbers from the EOB and Hospital Bill do not match up, the patient might be *balance billed*.

The Balance on the hospital bill should match the Patient Portion (or amount owed) on the EOB, for In-Network clients.

If they do not match and/or the Balance on your Hospital Bill matches the "Contractual Amount" or "Plan Discount" on your EOB, you may be getting balance billed.

For out-of-network healthcare services, the insurer's EOB will state this. It will also list the Gross Charges from the hospital and the amount that your insurance company paid the hospital or doctor's office, if any.

The hospital will then likely send the patient a separate bill for the difference between their Gross Charges and what the insurance company covered. This is the *Balance* in Balance Billing.

Even when patients go to an In-Network hospital for medical treatment, it is possible to have Out-of-Network charges.

It has become increasingly common for certain doctors or departments at in-network hospitals to be separate from the hospital and/or to not have an agreement with an insurance company, and to therefore be considered out-of-network.

For In-Network clients, fixing balance billing is relatively straightforward:

First confirm that you are being balance billed. The insurance company's representative should be able to walk through your charges and what you're responsible for and confirm whether this is the case.

Ask the representative the best way to talk to the hospital about getting the balance billing reversed. In-Network balance billing is forbidden in the contracts that insurance companies have with hospitals, so they will know how to correct this (and may do it for you).

If the insurance company did not offer to reach out to the hospital to correct the issue on your behalf, call the number on your hospital bill and let them know that you spoke to the insurance company, believe you're being balance billed, and politely request that they correct it.

Ask the hospital to send an updated and corrected bill. Once completed, make any payments you owe.

If the hospital that provided your treatment is out-of-network, you cannot use your insurance company for help.

Many states have laws prohibiting balance billing from out of network providers. A recent overview of state laws can be retrieved online via this website:

https://www.commonwealthfund.org/blog/2019/ state-efforts-protect-consumers-balance-billing

If your state has good out-of-network balance billing laws, you might be able to use those to reduce the amount you owe to the hospital, but you will first need to do some research and reading!

If you are confident that you understand your state law, you could call the hospital and politely state that you think you might have been balance billed against that state law.

You might need to ask to speak to someone about it, because

it is unlikely that the person answering the phone will be knowledgeable and/or have the authority to make changes to your bill.

With the right person on the phone, you should be able to walk through your argument in detail while they listen. If you are correct and you were *illegally* balance billed, the hospital should be able to easily correct it.

If your state does not have comprehensive balance billing laws, your path forward becomes more difficult.

You might be able to convince the biller that your portion of the current bill is large enough that it could cause you to go bankrupt, provided it's true.

You could also state that you would have gone In-Network if you had the chance, but that you did not have the option to do so. This positioning is particularly effective if you had required and/ or received emergency treatments and services.

You can work with the hospital - explaining the situation - to get them to agree to treat your bill as an In-Network amount.

If you need to talk to the hospital, keep in mind the following points:

> *Accepting your bill as an in-network claim will provide them with a fair rate for the services they provided.*

> *The current bill might bankrupt you (provided this is true), so the hospital will end up getting more money if they agree to treat your bill as an in-network claim.*

> *Because there are no laws or contractual obligations governing behavior, this can be a tricky and nuanced process.*

You will need to stay calm and patient and try to get the person on the other end of the line to see your point-of-view while understanding theirs.

There are two common types of billing errors.

An obvious one would be charges for services not provided, or for services you did not receive.

A more complex billing error might be hidden charges, which typically fall into one of two types: *unbundling* and *upcoding.*

The billing practice of unbundling means that the provider has taken a procedure that has a single code and then added additional codes for each of the "elements" of that procedure. For example, you may be billed for a panel of tests and then discover that elements have all been billed individually.

Upcoding refers to the biller putting a code on the bill for a service that is more complex and/or more costly than the services performed. A common example would be a visit to the ER. These are typically graded on a 1-5 scale, based on severity. A code for a level-5 visit might have been *upcoded* if the severity was level-4.

These situations are not easy to identify. You can look through an itemized bill line-by-line to try and spot billed services that you might not remember. If you are not sure of any such services, you can compare the bill with your Electronic Medical Record (EMR).

If you do not have an EMR, or need access to it online, you can call the hospital to ask them for it. In the U.S. the hospital is required by law to provide this to you, when requested by the patient.

To make things easier you can start with the biggest line items on your bill.
Medical codes and descriptions are confusing.

Use the Healthcare Blue Book and Google to search for HCPCS/CPT codes. If the most expensive items that you were billed for are correct, that bill is probably okay.

Sign up for a free trial of Find-A-Code to identify and track unbundling, or hidden charges. You can use the NCCI Edits

Validator (under Tools) to enter all the codes on your itemized bill.

Find-A-Code retrieves data from government-published CMS guidelines to detect code pairs that should not go together.

Upcoding is far more difficult.

The American College of Emergency Physicians has a good breakdown and explanation of what constitutes various ER visit levels, for example.

If you identify any billing errors, call the hospital's billing department to speak to someone about your bill. Then you will need to go through the items on the bill that you have identified as possible errors, one-at-a-time, and explain why you think they made an error.

Negotiating a hospital bill is not easy, but with enough knowledge and some research you should be able and achieve a better outcome and arrive at some amicable resolution

When you call the hospital or your insurance company about billing issues, they will be recording your call and taking notes about your conversation.

You might not be able to record the call, but you should also take notes of your conversations. Be sure to log the call dates and times, the name of the person you spoke with, what issues you discussed, etc.

Always be polite and patient, while being persistent.

It will be difficult for you to find an internal advocate in the billing department if you shout, use bad language, or start to get angry.

Try to become familiar with the person on the other end of the phone. Remember that he or she works in customer service, and that the representative you are speaking to was not the person or entity that sent you the bill you are trying to negotiate.

You may not achieve a desired answer, outcome, or conclusion right away. Remain polite, professional in your conversation and tone, and keep trying.

Do not give up!

*****

CHAPTER 11: IS THERE ANYBODY OUT THERE WHO WILL HELP ME?

Sometimes, despite your best efforts, medical bills are still too large to pay, and you may require help or relief. There are several options for you to consider.

At the time of writing, in 2022, the poverty line for a family of four was about $25,000 in annual household income.

Many hospitals offer financial assistance to people who have incomes 3-4x the federal poverty line. This implies that a family earning up to $100,000 per year might still qualify for financial aid from a hospital.

The process required for filing for hospital financial assistance is often time consuming and complicated.

Companies like Resolve - that you can find on the Internet - have created automated systems, helping their clients to collect the necessary files and information required for an application for hospital financial aid.

You can Google "[hospital name] financial assistance" to help you find out what information is available online or who to call to see if you qualify for any assistance offered and/or provided by your hospital.

You can also Google search to find out if you qualify for help from your state Medicaid office.

Medicaid eligibility is generally based on income levels. Your state's Medicaid office will determine whether you qualify.

Even if a healthcare or hospital procedure has already happened, you may still be able to qualify for *Retroactive Medicaid*. The US government allows for Medicaid coverage, retroactive for up to three months post-procedure.

Many states have a *Medically Needy* program.

The programs allow individuals with high medical expenses to reduce the income used to qualify for Medicaid by the amount they spend on their medical bills. Your best bet is to Google this, for the state where you live.

If your bill is for a child, you may qualify for your State's *Children's Health Insurance Program* (CHIP) funding.

Some pharmaceutical companies offer aid programs for people in financial need, to help pay for their drugs. Because drugs can be extremely expensive, *financial need* is loosely defined.

You can reach out directly to the pharmaceutical company that manufactures the drug, to ask if they offer any cost assistance programs to patients.

You can also conduct a Google search typing e.g., *medical bill charity for [treatment you received]*.

The results might show you charities that help with medical bills. Call and ask about getting help with medical bills. Even if the charity you call cannot assist you, they might be able to refer you to another agency.

You could start a *GoFundMe* campaign.

If you do so, you will need to market your campaign via your friends, family, and community.

More than 250,000 medical campaigns are posted per year (with over $650 million raised from those campaigns), according to GoFundMe.

For people just starting out using their website, they offer tips on how to run successful fundraising campaigns.

If you have exhausted every avenue for financial assistance, you might be able to apply for a *personal loan* from your bankers, for example. If this is your preferred route you need to remember that you will be responsible for making regular monthly payments to pay off the loan, plus interest.

Before taking out a personal loan, be sure to explore payment options with your hospital directly.

A hospital payment plan is often a much better alternative to a personal loan from a commercial lender. Hospital plans usually offer no- or low-interest loans, meaning you'll pay considerably less in the long run.

There are also various loan companies like LendingTree, Sofi, Earnest, Upstart, etc. to explore. This will allow you to shop around for the best interest rates on personal loans.

A final option is to take a chance, ignore the bills, and hope that they will *go away.*

This is not a recommended strategy.

Most hospitals will refer (or sell) delinquent accounts to collection agencies. The hospital (or collection agency) can take legal action to recover any money that might be due to them. They can apply for garnishments against your ongoing, earned income.

Any of these actions immediately above will likely hurt your credit score.

If you insist on taking this route, be sure to read the statute of limitations on debt collection for your state so that you will be familiar with the entire path you have elected to pursue.

If none of the suggestions above offer a solution, filing for bankruptcy might be the only option that remains.

You might wish to search and explore the National Association of Consumer Bankruptcy Attorneys (NACBA) website for a guide related to the pros and cons of bankruptcy, choosing an attorney, alternatives to bankruptcy, and more.

Many bankruptcy attorneys offer free consultations. This would allow you to discuss your situation with an expert, and to learn whether bankruptcy is the right option for you, or not.

*****

CHAPTER 11: IN CONCLUSION

There is no right to health care in the U.S. Constitution.

Congress has incrementally established health care rights through legislation, including the introduction of laws that created Medicare and Medicaid, the Emergency Medical Treatment and Active Labor Act, and the Affordable Care Act.

Article 25 of the United Nations Universal Declaration of Human Rights lists medical care as a basic human right.

The *right to health for all people* arguably means that everyone should have access to the health services they need, when and where they need them, without suffering financial hardship.

Really, no one should get sick and die just because they are poor, or because they cannot access the health services they need.

To be fair... despite the failings of the Great American Healthcare Billing Scam, as outlined in this book, many healthcare providers will see patients who are unable to pay and provide treatment anyway.

Many organizations - including U.S. hospitals - offer charitable programs and services for people who are unable to pay, zero interest payment plans for people who can afford to pay, and a variety of payment plans for people deemed wealthy enough to be able to pay *a big bill*, but perhaps unable to settle the entire bill, at once.

Philosophically, providing all citizens with access and a right to health care, is good for economic productivity. When people have access to health care, they live healthier lives and miss work less, allowing them to contribute more to the economy.

And, according to a Harvard study, despite spending far more on healthcare than other high-income nations, the U.S. scores poorly on many key health measures, including life expectancy, preventable hospital admissions, suicide, and maternal mortality.

Morally, a right to basic health care means that a government is obligated to do all within its means to ensure that medically necessary care is accessible and affordable to all.

Of course, the statement above does not imply that a government or physicians should be obligated to provide free face-lifts and tummy tucks on demand.

Essential elements of a right to health include non-discrimination, health facilities and services accessible to all, physical accessibility, economic accessibility (affordability) and information accessibility.

I wrote this book striving, as my core mission, to address the last two points above; namely economic, and information accessibility.

The current U.S. healthcare billing system applies costs to goods and/or services delivered based on nothing but a thumb-suck, often more affectionately referred to as *a sucker price* (which no one pays).

Usually, merchants will sell the services or products they produce at a retail price that is based on their costs, including time and materials.

In a free market environment, the market will accept or reject the price of the goods and/or services. If the value does not match the price, merchants have options. They can either adjust their prices, or eventually go out of business.

In the U.S. healthcare system, the cabals that collectively manage the system - government, healthcare providers, drug companies, insurance companies, etc. - colluded to create a multi-tiered system: one for the rich, another for the insured middle class, a different system for the uninsured, one for the poor, and yet another one for incarcerated people (who are wards of the state).

Arguably, *the rich* can purchase whatever they want.

The insured, under-insured, and uninsured people - i.e., most people (or the shrinking middle class) - are the people most often at the mercy of the Great American Healthcare Billing Scam.

The poor will often rely on charity out of necessity.

Incarcerated people in the U.S. have access to most medical services.

In both these examples immediately above, the taxpayers would foot the bill, either via charitable donations, or directly by paying taxes on their earnings.

That large middle group, as described a few paragraphs above, represents the target audience for this book.

If I were to help just one person avoid bankruptcy, it would have been worth my time and effort to write this book!

If, because of this book, a few people manage to successfully negotiate exorbitant medical bills - and get these adjusted or discounted to amounts deemed more affordable to them - then my time and effort was also suitably rewarded.

And finally, I did not write this book for any personal financial or other reward.

As I have done with previous written works, I order author's copies in bulk at discounted prices. I pay for these purchases with my own money i.e., out-of-pocket. I offer my books to people in exchange for a donation. Whatever amount they can afford as a donation, determines the price.

I donate 100% of the gross revenue for my book sales to Memory Trees Corporation, a registered public charity. You can learn more about our No Poverty projects via our website: memorytrees.co.

*****

CHAPTER 12: TWO YEARS LATER...THE GRAND FINALE?!

Over a few months, as medical bills kept trickling in, the total amount billed for my medical misfortune edging ever closer to $200,000.

The last *invoice* I received was only mailed on March 27th, 2024, nearly two years to the date of the start of my adventure.

I italicized the word *invoice* above, because it was actually a final notice from a debt collector. Despite me having received zero, nada, zilch communication or invoices for the original ambulance trip to the ER on March 26th, 2022, I received a demand letter because I had never paid the bill.

The sender - a collections agency - kindly offered me 30 days to dispute the debt. They wrote: "Call or write to us by May 2, 2024, to dispute all or part of the debt. If you do not, we will assume that all our information is correct."

I wrote back on April 5, 2024:

> *I received the enclosed notification from your organization today, April 5, 2024. It includes the references "you received*

medical service" and the date "03/26/2022". Based on these two aforesaid references, I assume that the "service" might refer to a 5 mile journey via ambulance that the City provided, from my home to XXXXXXX ER on that date?

I have not previously received an invoice or any communication related to any services delivered.

The City should have billed my insurer at the time. I had provided my insurance card at the time of the ambulance pickup at my house. They would have processed the invoice and paid their portion (as applicable). Then they would have sent me an Explanation of Benefits indicating my portion due for payment/negotiation (if any).

Florida Chapter 627 Statute 736*: "If a person has an emergency medical condition and receives emergency services from an out-of-network provider or facility **the most they can bill is the patient's in-network cost-sharing amount.**" A patient also cannot be balance-billed for emergency services. Pursuant to this same section, a Florida "person or institution lawfully rendering [ambulance/emergency] treatment **may only charge the insurer and injured party a reasonable amount** for the services and supplies rendered."*

Today, I tried to log into my previous insurer's account online. It appears as if they are no longer active and/or still in business (see attached info).

*Due to: (a) the extraordinary length of time that has lapsed since the service date, (b) NO PREVIOUS communication/ invoice received from The City related to this service, and (c) because and amount of $214.03 (Medicare rate 09102 for ambulance services paid at 100% of the fee) represents a "reasonable amount" (as per FL Statute 736 above) that my insurer might have paid in full settlement, **I will personally not make any payment and consider this debt as canceled.***

An amount of $738.85 is therefore still outstanding as of April 2024, and I offered to pay $0.

If they were to write back saying they would accept $214.03 in full and final settlement of the amount due, I would be willing to pay that lesser amount. Otherwise, I will simply pay nothing, and wait patiently for them to *go away* - a most likely outcome for a City-generated demand for payment for medical services that are arguably already paid for by homeowners and residents via their property taxes.

*****

The largest bills were the hospital invoices totalling more than $100,000 for my in-patient lodging and services for a few days and nights. Even though I had offered to settle these bills for $20,000, the hospital kindly ended up forgiving the entire amount invoiced.

The $100,000 had been split into two invoices of about $60,000 and $40,000, respectively. The larger one was forgiven in 2023, while the smaller amount was still showing as outstanding in account - but with *$0 due now* - for another few months.

When I logged into my account in January 2024 to check in, the entire account balance showed $0, meaning the hospital had written off the entire debt as unpaid, or as settled via their charity, etc. I am not sure and I did not inquire as to why or when the outstanding balance was zeroed out.

I was delighted to learn that $100,000 owed to one provider - for the two largest amounts invoiced - had been changed to $0. The debt had been forgiven somehow, over time, and for whatever reasons.

Of course the reason for the debt forgiveness might be as a result of my request to reduce the amount owing, but I cannot be certain of that because they never communicated with me after I had submitted my offer.

*****

I settled several of the out-of-network doctors' invoices for between $250-350 each, respectively.

Three of these above invoices were for ER doctors who each billed me about $2,500. I used the Medicare rate plus 10% as an offer of payment in full and final settlement, and they all accepted that payment and *closed the file*.

Another two were "doctors" who each billed me about $3,000 - via the same billing service - for consulting services they had delivered to me while I was in hospital.

One of these providers is a complete mystery to me. I have no recollection of her consulting with me as her patient.

The other, who my wife and I affectionately named *Betty Short Skirts*, was a short, voluptuous lady who wore dresses or skirts of a length that were arguably not work appropriate... since nursing often requires lifting, bending over, reaching for items, etc.

Primarily for this particular dress-length reason, I remember speaking with *Dr. Betty* a couple of times, unlike my lack of memory regarding her colleague.

I sent their billing service two checks for $250 each, offering the *payment in full and final settlement* for their two invoices totalling more than $6,000.

The billing service returned my checks, and included a letter stating that my reference to the Medicare rate plus 10% was outdated. The new (or current at the time) Medicare rate plus my offered 10% would be $300.

I regarded their pricing information as a counter-offer to my original offer, and sent them two checks for $300 each, also marked as *payment in full and final settlement.*

For clarity, any check payments I sent via mail included a letter from me stating that, "Your deposit of the enclosed check indicates acceptance of my payment in full and final settlement of the amount invoiced."

I never heard anything further from the five doctors described above.

The total of their five invoices - about $13,500 - was therefore settled with five separate payments, for a total amount of $1,350.

For those of you who might be keeping track, and as per previous examples provided earlier, it appears as if most medical healthcare billing scam invoices could be settled for about 10% of the invoiced amounts.

My medical insurer - which has at the time of writing this appears to have gone out of business - rejected the surgeon's bill for the investigative laparoscopy he had performed.

The reason for nonpayment was that the provider - as is custom for planned, future, non-medical procedures - should have requested preauthorization from the patient's insurer prior to delivery of any services.

At the time they rejected the surgeon's bill, the insurer advised the billing service that they may apply for approval in arrears, or after the fact, and asked them to submit that request for approval for a negotiated (insured) amount.

The surgeon and/or his billing service did not reply and as a result of their noncompliance and/or lack of response, they received no reimbursement for their previously invoiced services.

I know this to be true because the insurer sent me an Explanation of Benefits statement for every claim they received from in- and out-of- network providers for services they claimed to have provided.

Some invoices that were sent to my insurance company for out-of-network services that were rejected by my insurer simply *went away*, and we never heard from them again.

*****

I guess it might be reasonable to imagine that The Great American Healthcare Billing Scam is so fat with profits; corrupt to the core in terms of aggressive over-billing for non-delivered and/ or poor services; administratively inefficient; and - perhaps most importantly - squeezes enough juice from the available oranges to have to worry about nuisance, ever-questioning hagglers like me?

To date, two years later, I have paid about $10,000 of the original $200,000 in total billings, out of pocket. Although it is possible that there might still be invoices trickling in, like my local city's EMS bill that arrived - as a final demand - in April 2024, I am comfortable that the ordeal is now firmly in the past, and finished.

Regrettably, one day you might have a similar story to tell.

You will have four basic options to consider: (a) pay (your portion of) the bill if you are able to do so; (b) negotiate a fair price and pay those bills, or the patient portion determined by your insurer if you are insured; (c) ignore all the bills and hope they go away; and/ or (d) pay nothing, and declare bankruptcy.

That is my story.

I hope your story, when you share it one day, will be a better recollection of events and circumstances, than mine!

GLOSSARY

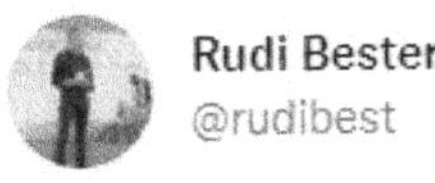

Replying to @Linny_Pin99

I was in hospital last month for the first time in my life. Their "standard care protocols" will literally kill you.

I discharged myself, walked out, went home and have now recovered.

Do not go to hospital if you are able to avoid doing so!

7:33 AM · May 5, 2022 · Twitter for Android

A tweet (reflecting frustration with the "system") following my personal experience, post-hospitalization.

*****

Service	Charge	Discount	Paid	pay	Amount	Deductible	Notes
EMERGENCY DEPT VISIT HIGH SEVERITY&THREAT FUNCJ (99285)	$2,054.00	$0.00	$0.00	$0.00	$0.00	$238.04	Reimbursement is based on the regulations under the No Surprises Act o r applicable state law. Member is not responsible and cannot be balanc ed billed for covered out of network services beyond allowed amount. F or more information on open negotiations and dispute resolution please visit: https://brighthealthcare.com/provider/federal-no-surprises-act
ECG ROUTINE ECG W/LEAST 12 LDS I&R ONLY (93010)	$96.00	$0.00	$0.00	$0.00	$0.00	$10.87	Reimbursement is based on the regulations under the No Surprises Act o r applicable state law. Member is not responsible and cannot be balanc ed billed for covered out of network services beyond allowed amount. F or more information on open negotiations and dispute resolution please visit: https://brighthealthcare.com/provider/federal-no-surprises-act
Total	$2,150.00	$0.00	$0.00	$0.00	$0.00	$248.91	

An example of a subcontractor bill for $2,054 discounted to $238.04 by the insurer, based on the U.S. Federal No Surprises Act (more info below).

Provider Arbitration pursuant to the Federal No Surprises Act:

If this claim is subject to the Federal No Surprises Act, the paid amount is the lesser of billed charges or the qualifying payment amount for this item or service, which is calculated in accordance with the No Surprises Act and implementing regulations.

The qualifying payment amount also applies for purposes of the recognized amount (or, in the case of air ambulance services, for calculating the participant's, beneficiary's, or enrollee's cost sharing).

Payments are made in compliance with the Federal No Surprises Act or applicable state law.

The member is not responsible and cannot be balance billed for covered out of network services beyond allowed amounts.

*****

Pre-authorization and Provider Tax Identification Number:

Service	Charge	Discount	Paid	pay	Amount	Deductible	Notes
SBSQ HOSPITAL CARE/DAY 35 MINUTES (99233)	$746.00	$0.00	$0.00	$0.00	$0.00	$0.00	WE HAVE NO RECORD OF PRE-AUTHORIZATION FOR THE FACILITY PORTION OF THI S STAY/SERVICE. UPON RECEIPT OF THE FACILITY'S CLAIM, THE FACILITY WIL L BE ADVISED TO OBTAIN RETRO-AUTHORIZATION. THIS CLAIM WILL BE DELAYED UNTIL AUTHORIZATION IS OBTAINED.
SBSQ HOSPITAL CARE/DAY 35 MINUTES (99233)	$746.00	$0.00	$0.00	$0.00	$0.00	$0.00	WE HAVE NO RECORD OF PRE-AUTHORIZATION FOR THE FACILITY PORTION OF THI S STAY/SERVICE. UPON RECEIPT OF THE FACILITY'S CLAIM, THE FACILITY WIL L BE ADVISED TO OBTAIN RETRO-AUTHORIZATION. THIS CLAIM WILL BE DELAYED UNTIL AUTHORIZATION IS OBTAINED.
Total	$1,492.00	$0.00	$0.00	$0.00	$0.00	$0.00	

An example of a bill rejected by an insurer because they had no "record of pre-authorization" for services delivered.

Neither the patient, nor the hospital, would likely have been aware of the insurer's pre-authorization requirements, according to the patient's medical insurance plan.

*****

Comparing an insurer's Explanation of Benefits ("EOB") to a hospital's Itemized Bill:

Service	Charge	Discount	Paid	pay	Amount	Deductible
undefined (undefined)	$470.00	$0.00	$0.00		$0.00	
undefined (undefined)	$470.00	$0.00	$0.00		$0.00	
undefined (undefined)	$275.00	$0.00	$0.00		$0.00	
undefined (undefined)	$4,150.00	$0.00	$0.00	$0.00	$0.00	$0.00
undefined (undefined)	$707.00	$0.00	$0.00		$0.00	
undefined (undefined)	$12,793.00	$0.00	$0.00	$0.00	$0.00	$0.00
undefined (undefined)	$1,764.00	$0.00	$0.00		$0.00	
undefined (undefined)	$5,496.00	$0.00	$0.00		$0.00	
undefined (undefined)	$294.00	$0.00	$0.00	$0.00	$0.00	$0.00
undefined (undefined)	$143.00	$0.00	$0.00		$0.00	
undefined (undefined)	$751.00	$0.00	$0.00		$0.00	
Total	$34,630.00	$0.00	$0.00	$0.00	$0.00	$0.00

A snapshot of an Explanation of Benefits (EOB) above from an insurer with no descriptions and codes. Insured patients cannot use this for reconciliation, comparison, or verification purposes.

```
040322    1  30    VENIPUNC  51048874        0.00      0.00
040322    1  45    3MLEVEL   43022557     4214.00      0.00
040322    1  45    ER STATI  43034958        0.00      0.00
040322    1  45    3MIV INF  43035005      682.00      0.00
040322    1  51    CT ABD P  53473518    12793.00      0.00
040322    1  68    MORPHINE  54062211       43.00      0.00
040322    1  68    ONDANSET  54336789       40.00      0.00
040322    1  G     ROOM  37  61600102     3198.00      0.00
040422    1  23    FAMOTIDI  54302559      122.00      0.00
040422    1  30    BMP       51000057      645.00      0.00
040422    1  30    CBC AUTO  51009579      470.00      0.00
040422    1  30    SPEC COL  51018851       86.00      0.00
040422    1  30    VENIPUNC  51048874        0.00      0.00
040422   -1  30    VENIPUNC  51048874        0.00      0.00
040422    1  68    MORPHINE  54062211       43.00      0.00
040422    2  68    POT CHL   54075478     1056.00      0.00
040422   -2  68    POT CHL   54075478    -1056.00      0.00
040422    1  68    POT CHL   54360276       43.00      0.00
040422    1  G     ROOM  37  61600102     3198.00      0.00
```

A snapshot of "the same" bill (as illustrated above), but this time, an Itemized Bill from the hospital with services descriptions and codes.

*****

A subcontractor's bill for out-of-network services provided to the patient:

of Service	Charge	Discount	Paid	pay	Amount	Deductible	Notes
INITIAL HOSPITAL CARE/DAY 70 MINUTES (99223)	$1,449.00	$0.00	$0.00	$0.00	$0.00	$0.00	CONFIRMS THAT BHPCO REVIEWED AND APPRVED SERVICES RENDERED BY A NON-PARTICIPATING PROVIDER ARE NOT COVERED. IF PROVIDER IS IN NETWORK UNDER A DIFFERENT TAX IDENTIFICATION/NPI NUMBER , THE CLAIM MUST BE RESUBMITTED WITH THAT TAX IDENTIFICATION/NPI NUMBE R FOR CONSIDERATION.**** PLEASE REFER TO THE LIMITATIONS/EXCLUSIONS SE CTION OF THE CERTIFICATE OF COVERAGE. Services rendered by an out-of-network provider are not covered.
Total	$1,449.00	$0.00	$0.00	$0.00	$0.00	$0.00	

An Explanation of Benefits from the insurance company notifying the claimant that "out-of-network" providers are not covered by their insurance policy.

They advise that if the provider has a different tax identification number, the provider may resubmit the claim under that number.

Otherwise, the patient will be responsible for paying the bill.

*****

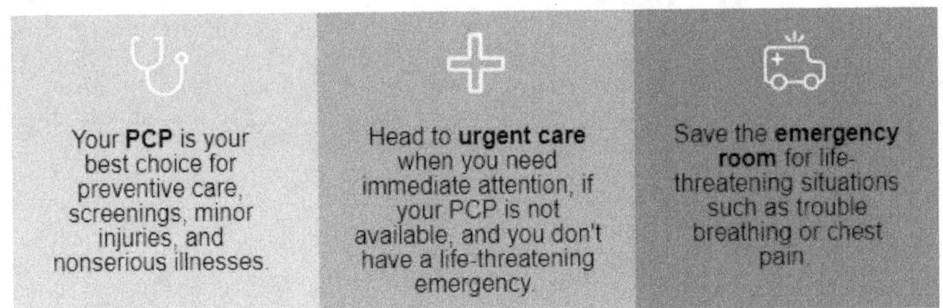

Recommended for patients: Primary Care Physician (PCP) is for everyday consultations, urgent care for emergencies, and ER for life-threatening emergencies.

Below are two large hospital bills as per the medical provider's website. Note that the amount has been adjusted, but in this example the patient does not yet know why, or whether this adjustment is correct.

The patient will not know what the actual amount due for payment is, until the hospital receives the final reconciliation statement from the patient's insurance company.

The patient might incorrectly assume that he or she will be liable for 10% of the Total Charges, at this time.

Account Activity

Total Charges:	$66,202.00
Ins. Payments & Adjustments:	$59,581.80
Insurance Pending:	$0.00
Patient Payments:	$0.00
Current Account Balance:	$0.00
Monthly Payment Amount:	$0.00
I Owe:	$0.00
Insurance for this Account	contact us

Account Activity

Total Charges:	$34,630.00
Ins. Payments & Adjustments:	$31,167.00
Insurance Pending:	$0.00
Patient Payments:	$0.00
Current Account Balance:	$0.00
Monthly Payment Amount:	$0.00
I Owe:	$0.00
Insurance for this Account	contact us

*****

BOOKS BY THIS AUTHOR

Walking On Water

This is the personal life story of Rudi Bester.

Entrepreneur. Investor. Charitable Benefactor. Businessman. Father. Husband. YouTube Content Creator. Author.

"When I was young, I was very poor. After a lifetime of hard work and commitment, I am no longer young." This line, probably more than any other from the book, summarizes Rudi's life best. With no parental guidance, a missing and/or broken family structure, one has to learn survival techniques by oneself. Failure is a good teacher, success less so. Follow Rudi on a path of being unwittingly born into poverty and homelessness, across different countries, as he learned survival and financial sustainability skills, en route.

I trust that Walking on Water will be an enjoyable read... but one that also provides a little real-world financial education!

Mergers & Acquisitions

This short research paper provides an easy-to-read research study and overview of M&A as a corporate strategy. Business leaders may often ponder why mergers and acquisitions are so popular as a corporate growth strategy? And perhaps why the published failure rates of M&A are seemingly so high?

Perhaps whether the primary purpose of embarking on a

corporate M&A strategy is focused on delivering investor and/ or shareholder return on investment, i.e. wealth creation? "M&A" strives to explore the logic and reason behind questions business leaders often ponder when pursuing a corporate growth strategy via M&A.

Not all of the above will be viewed as having been successful, but objectively, measuring success depends on the real reason - or success metrics - in place to determine why an executive management team embarked on a corporate acquisition strategy in the first place.

Whether popular, or successful, a strategy pursuing mergers and/ or acquisitions is as old as business itself. I hope that you will enjoy reading this short research paper as much as I had enjoyed writing it!